THE BEST EXERCISES YOU'VE NEVER HEARD OF

Published by Price World Publishing
1300 W Belmont Ave Ste 20G
Chicago, IL 60657-3200
www.PriceWorldPublishing.com

Copyright © 2012 by Nick Nilsson & BetterU, Inc.

ISBN: 9781932549805
eBook ISBN: 9781936910182
Library of Congress Control Number: 2012936937

Printing by Sheridan Books
Printed in the United States of America
10 9 8 7 6 5 4 3 2 1

For information about discounts for bulk purchases, please contact info@priceworldpublishing.com.

THE BEST EXERCISES YOU'VE NEVER HEARD OF

NICK NILSSON

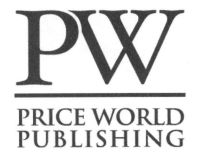

PRICE WORLD
PUBLISHING

Welcome to "The Best Exercises You've Never Heard Of!"

From:
Nick Nilsson

Let's be honest: **normal training is boring, and quite often ineffective!**

THAT is where I come in.

The unique exercises in this book will help you take your muscular development to a whole new level. You'll learn exercises that cover ALL aspects of your body: chest, back, thighs, arms, shoulders, you name it.

Take some time to flip through all of the exercises and try out the ones you like. You will be AMAZED at how well they hit your entire body and how FAST they will accelerate your development.

Enjoy!

TABLE OF CONTENTS

ABDOMINALS

DUMBBELL PALLOF PRESS

This is a very good variation of the Pallof Press. The Pallof Press is done using a single cable handle, using it to rotate your torso directly to the side. Start with the handle in against your body, then push it out. When it comes out and away from the body, your core functions to prevent that rotation.

Normally, that exercise is done using just a single cable handle.

The version I'm going to show you here also uses a dumbbell for extra resistance. You'll be holding it up in addition to resisting the cable's rotation.

Grab the cable handle and pick up the dumbbell so that you're clasping it with both hands. Take a step out to the side with one leg. You can set your feet in a staggered position or directly in line with each other.

Start with the dumbbell held in at your abdomen.

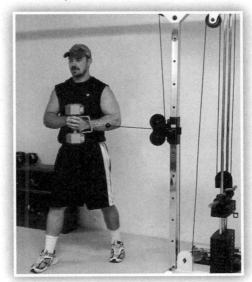

Now, keeping your core TIGHT, extend your arms, moving the dumbbell and cable away from your body. THIS is the money part of the exercise. The cable is pulling you to the right, and you have to resist that rotation while the dumbbell is trying to pull your arms down, which you ALSO have to fight.

This double resistance places a tremendous demand on the entire core musculature.

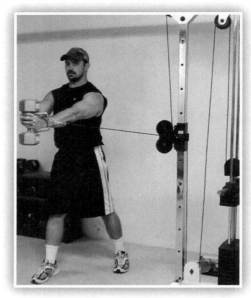

Perform 4 to 6 repetitions on one side. Set the dumbbell down before switching to the other side.

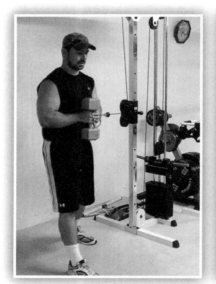 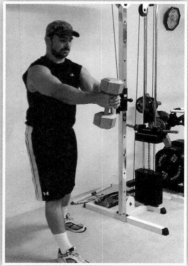

If you've never done the Pallof Press, try it without the dumbbell first. THEN start with a light dumbbell. This is a nice variation of the exercise that is going to really light up your midsection.

BAR AND BENCH TRANSITION PLANKS

I f you're interested in flatter abs and a stronger core, the plank is one of the key exercises you should be doing. Once the normal abdominal plank gets too easy, you've got a variety of options to make it more challenging, more interesting and more effective.

This is one of those options!

This is a nice variation of the plank that involves dynamic transitions between two different plank positions: forearm and straight-arm planks. The benefit lies in the moment of transition between the two positions.

You can do this type of dynamic plank on the floor, but I prefer to do it on a flat bench with a barbell set in the power rack (or another bar set at the right height, be it a Smith machine or even the handle of another machine). I'll tell you why this is effective once I've shown you the exercise.

So first, set the bar a little above the level of the bench and set the bench about four or five feet away from the bar. Where you place it will depend on how tall you are; you'll need to adjust it to get the spacing right.

Set your forearms on the bench, and then hook your toes over the bar, keeping your body straight and stiff.

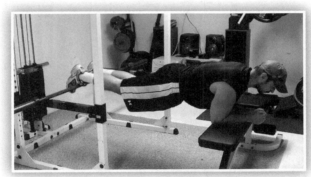

Now, the reason I use the bar is that I find when doing the plank on the ground with the toes on the floor, it increases leg/hip flexor contribution to the stabilization of the core. When you hook the toes over a bar, it takes some of that contribution away and focuses more on the core for the stabilizing tension.

This will immediately make the plank harder to do.

The next step is to transition to a straight-arm plank:

Lean on the right arm, then set your left hand on the bench.

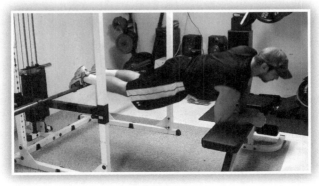

Straighten your left arm, then set your right hand flat on the bench. At multiple points during this transition, you're basically planking on one arm.

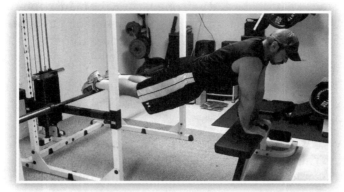

Repeat on the opposite side, setting your left forearm on the bench while bending your right arm.

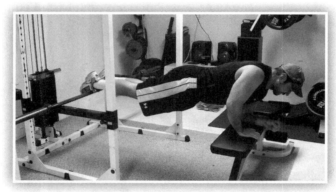

Now you're back with your forearms flat on the bench.

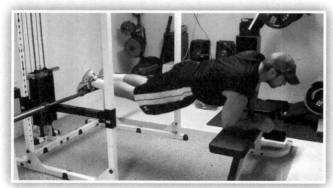

Repeat the maneuver until you can no longer support your body in the plank position.

Now, this one sounds simple but is actually surprisingly tough to do. Transitioning while the majority of the tension goes through one side and your toes are hooked over the bar instead of set on the floor puts a whole different tension on the core.

If you're new to the plank, this is not the version you should jump in and start with. If you're already familiar with the plank, you will really enjoy this variation and how it targets the oblique muscles and deep transverse abdominus muscles with the dynamic repositioning of the arms.

DUMBBELL AND ANKLE WEIGHT CRAWLING

Dumbbell Crawling is an exercise you may not be familiar with. It is a KILLER abdominal exercise and all you need is a pair of dumbbells and a floor. Basically, you're holding the dumbbells in your hands and crawling forward, moving your hands and feet in alternating steps.

The "easy" version is done just with dumbbells (and you work up to some pretty sizeable dumbbells). I've gone a step further and added in ankle weights, just to make it REALLY fun. When you're looking at this one, keep in mind you can do it without the ankle weights as well, if you don't have them.

The addition of ankle weights targets the lower portion of the core more so than just the dumbbells.

Make sure you have an open stretch of floor, at least 10 to 12 feet in length. Lean down and set your hands on the dumbbell handles (your ankle weights should already be on).

Now move the right dumbbell forward and your left foot forward. Your right foot and left hand will be supporting your body as you lift your right hand up and left leg up. This puts GREAT cross-tension on the entire core.

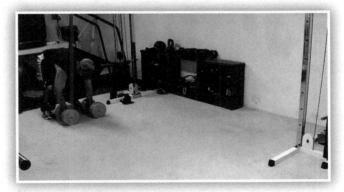

Now step the other opposing pair forward.

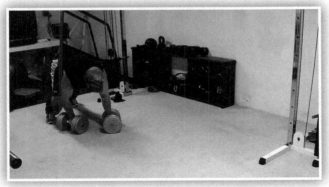

And continue across the floor in this fashion.

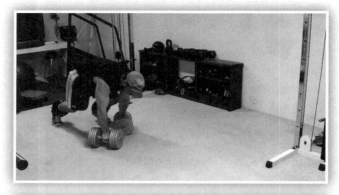

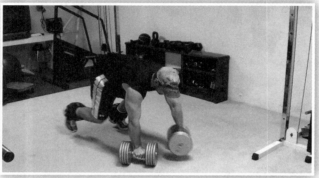

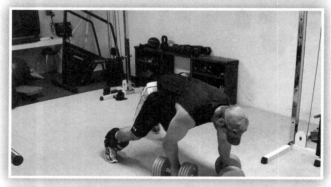

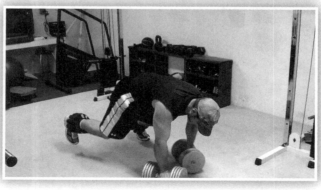

Go as far forward as you can, then walk yourself BACKWARDS. This is actually harder than going forward, since you have to pull the dumbbell back.

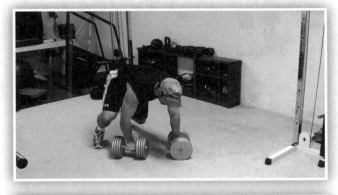

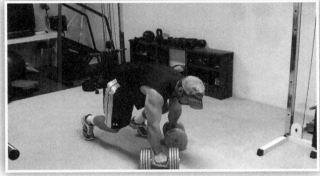

Keep going for as long as you can, until you have a hard time moving the dumbbells forward or you nearly fall down.

This is one of my favorite core training exercises. It's very simple to do and very effective in terms of functionality of the core.

LOCKOUT ONE SHOULDER
BARBELL SQUATS

T his exercise is going to KILL your core...in a good way.

It's a partial-range version of the One Shoulder Barbell Squat exercise, which I normally would do in a full range of motion.

Having the bar supported on just one shoulder is incredibly good core training. It forces a lot of stabilizing work in the core, while still giving your legs some decent work as well. The full-range version of this exercise is tough (definitely check that out at the link above). This partial-range version takes the weight used in the exercise to the extreme.

If you've got a very strong core, you can work with this partial range one right away (start lighter than what I'm using-I've been around the block with this exercise). You can work up to some substantial weights.

First, set the rails in the rack to about four to six inches below lockout squat height—you can play with the height a bit with just the unloaded bar on the rails to get it to where you want it. Now put a barbell pad on the bar or fold up a towel and put it over your shoulder for padding.

Stand under the center of the bar facing the side of the rack and brace the bar on one shoulder, in the groove between the trapezius and the deltoid. Grab the bar in front of you with both hands. Set your feet out fairly wide to increase your base of support; since the bar is on one side of your body, you have to extend the base of support to perform the exercise with power and stability.

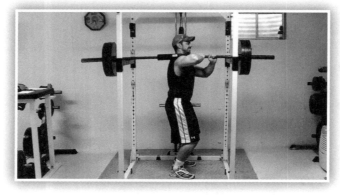

Now stand up.

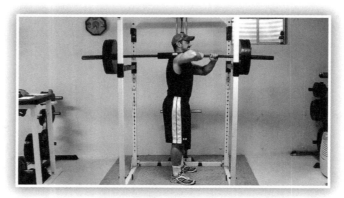

Repeat for 3 to 5 reps on one side, and then switch.

I also recommend keeping your elbow fairly high to provide greater stability for the barbell. Raising the arm like this keeps the bar in the shoulder groove.

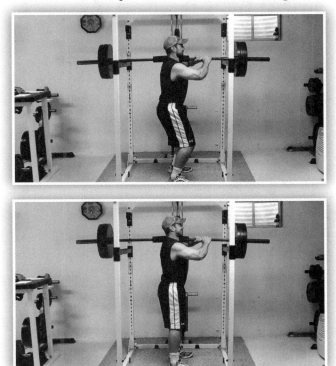

Do your reps on the other side.

That's it! Simple exercise but just standing up with that amount of weight on the bar on just one side of your body puts tremendous tension on the core.

I'm using 315 pounds in the pictures above.

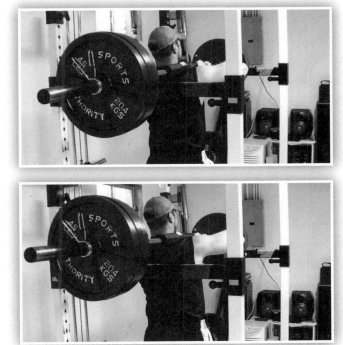

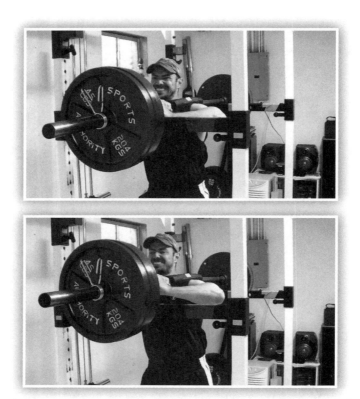

This is a challenging variation of a very challenging exercise! It's a total body movement that will really do a number on your core, upper body and legs; pretty much everything.

LOWER AB PLANKS IN RACK

The Plank is one of the best and most simple abdominal exercises you can do. If you're not familiar with the Plank, you hold your body in a horizontal position with your forearms and toes on the floor, maintaining a straight body position for as long as possible.

It's a great exercise you can do anywhere.

THIS exercise is a version of that. I've got it set up in the rails of a power rack, but you can very easily do it between two benches if you don't have a rack to work with (or a bench for your forearms and something else a few feet off the ground to hook your feet over—you'll see what I mean).

To do this one in the rack, set the rails a few feet off the ground, then stand facing one side. Set your forearms (near the elbow) on the rail, and then hook your feet on the other rail. Now just hold your body in that position, keeping your body just a bit bent (not completely straight like the floor version. Because your knees are lower, you need to keep some bend in your hips to keep pressure off the lower back) and as stable as you can.

I find the angle of the body and legs puts a lot more tension on the lower abdominal area than the standard floor plank.

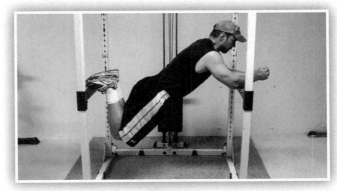

It's easier to see the bend in the hips from this view. Keeping the hips bent is really important. If you straighten the body, you'll immediately get a lot of stress on the lower back.

Once again, though, this is a nice exercise for targeting the lower abdominal area and you can do it on benches or anything else that you can set your forearms and feet on.

ON-DUMBBELL ABDOMINAL ROLL-OUTS

T he Ab Roll-Out is a powerful exercise for strengthening the core. But what if you don't have a wheel or other apparatus for performing the exercise?

No problem! You can just use a dumbbell, and it doesn't even have to have loose plates. I like to use at least an 85 lb dumbbell; you can use more but the number of plates will help make the exercise more comfortable. You'll see why.

Kneel in front of the dumbbell and set your hands on top of the plates.

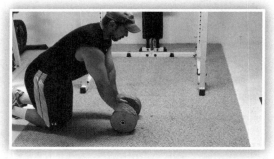

Now start rolling forward on the dumbbell, keeping your hands on the plates.

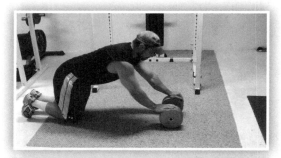

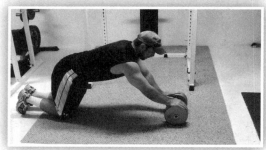

Keep going until you're fully stretched out . You'll be resting pretty much on your forearms very near the elbows at the end.

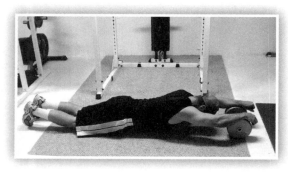

From there, just pull yourself back up into the starting position, rolling the dumbbell back.

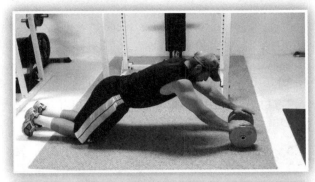

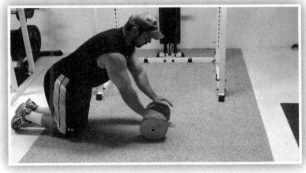

The great thing with this one is that you not only get the basic roll-out exercise, you also get the weight of the dumbbell to work against! Being round, it isn't really a LOT of resistance, but it does add up as you do more reps.

ONE SIDE LOADED BARBELL SQUATS

This exercise is a very simple but VERY effective way to strongly hit your core. It looks like squat, stands like a squat, and IS a squat but it doesn't work the legs!

Pretty simply, you're going to just load ONE side of the bar with 25 to 45 pounds or so. Start at the lighter end until you get an idea of how the balance on this exercise works.

It's best to do this exercise in a squat rack. Load the bar, set it across your upper back/traps as you normally would for squats. Hold on TIGHTLY, then step back.

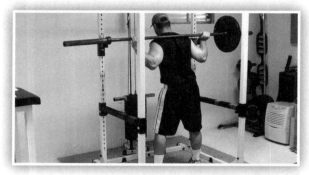

The first thing you'll notice, of course, is the weight pulling down on the right side. Pull hard with your left arm to keep the bar locked in place on your back; the goal is to keep the bar horizontal while you're squatting.

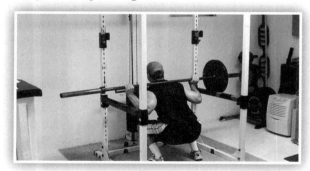

From there, it's basically a matter of squatting! Go down as far as you can and then push back up. The uneven load on the bar will force your side core area to contract strongly.

It's a great way to build side core strength and power.

Do all your reps on one side, and then set the weight on the other side of the bar and go again:

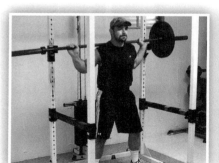
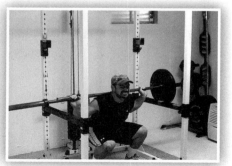

This one will really challenge your core strength.

PERPENDICULAR BAR
HANGING LEG RAISES

This is a simple twist on the regular hanging leg raise exercise. Instead of hanging from the bar facing forward, you will instead turn 90 degrees so that your body is perpendicular to the bar, then you'll do hanging leg raises.

How is this different, you might ask?

The answer is that the close-in hand position actually allows you to better target the oblique muscles while doing the leg raise. Normally, when you do the hanging leg raise exercise, your hands are at least a foot or more apart for stability. With this version, you're using a baseball-bat-type grip so your hands are directly overhead. This puts the arms at an angle to your torso, which automatically involves the obliques.

You can also bring your legs up in a twisting movement to further accentuate the oblique involvement, which I will also show below.

Since I'm doing these in the rack, I have my hands set a bit back from the center point to allow room for my legs to come up. This is more of a knee raise, because of the space constraints-if you have enough room around your chin-up bar, you can do a full leg raise with the legs straighter. This version works really well though, too.

To start, grip the bar like a baseball bat, and then hang.

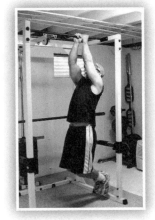

Now, start raising the legs/knees. Be sure to start the movement with flexion at the abdominals, not just hinging at the hips.

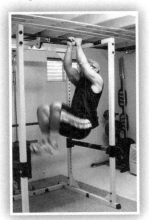

I like to come all the way up until my feet are by the bar and my upper body is almost horizontal.

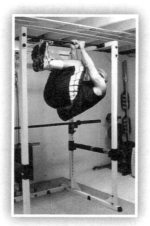

You can also come up twisting, with your knees tilted to one side.

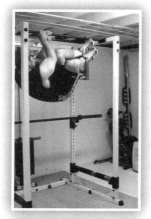

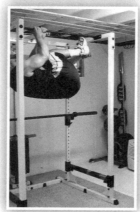

This is great oblique work and all it takes is a simple positioning change in the hanging leg-raise grip.

PUSH-PULLS, A.K.A. THE AB RIPPER

This is one of my very favorite "secret weapon" total-torso training exercises. It covers pretty much every major part in your upper body in just one movement (or should I say TWO movements in one!).

It's a relatively simple-looking concept on the surface: you'll be doing a single-arm dumbbell bench press while at the same time doing a single arm cable pulldown/row.

As you're pushing the dumbbell UP, you're pulling the cable DOWN, so you're hitting the two biggest parts of the upper body in one shot (including biceps on the pull and triceps on the press, along with aspects of the shoulders on both).

What you might not see at first glance is the INCREDIBLE core cross-tension you'll get when you execute a push and a pull. You see, in order to stabilize the core while doing two opposing movements, your deep core muscles (oblique and transversus) will be pushed to the limit.

This is honestly one of THE best core exercises I've ever come up with, never mind all the other upper body stuff going on. It's going to develop incredible core strength without any hint of a crunch or sit-up.

I can promise you, if you've never done heavy cross-core tension training before, your deep abdominal muscles will be feeling it for DAYS. So start with more moderate weights than I'm using in the demo here and work up to it.

Here's how to do it:

First, you'll need a flat bench, a high pulley with a single handle, and a dumbbell. Set the bench lengthwise next to the high pulley and set the dumbbell in front of the bench.

I'm using a 95 lb dumbbell and about 120 pounds on the pulley. You'll need to do a little practice to get the weight balance right for yourself. The dumbbell should be something you can control pretty easily. Balance the pulldown part in accordance with the dumbbell you're pressing.

Pick up the dumbbell with your right hand, sit on the end of the bench and rest the dumbbell on your right thigh.

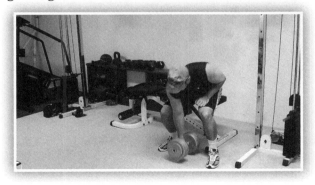

Now reach up and grab the single cable handle with your left hand.

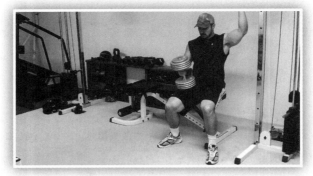

Scoot forward off the bench and lay back so only your shoulders are on the bench.

Your upper arm should be resting on the bench and your left shoulder will be stretched up and off the bench. Get ready to push and pull!

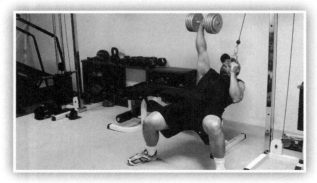

Start the press and at the same time start the pull. They should be simultaneous. THIS is where you'll start to feel the incredible cross-tension in the core!

With the pulldown/row, you'll want to keep your elbow in close to your body; not a wide-grip row position, more like a close-grip row.

Press all the way up and pull down as far as you can.

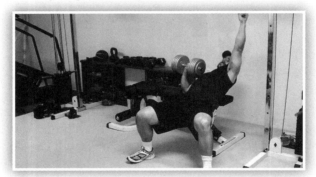

Now just lower the dumbbell and let the cable go up and repeat! I like to keep to lower reps on this one; the core responds better to lower reps and resistance. So, as I mentioned, start with moderate resistance but definitely work your way up.

On each rep, you can rest your upper arm on the bench, similar to a floor dumbbell bench press. It's not a full-range press, but you'll find you won't really care by the time you've done a set.

To finish the exercise, let your upper arm rest on the bench and release the cable handle.

Reach over and stabilize the dumbbell with the left hand. Then just shift your legs around to a kneeling position, and lower the dumbbell to the floor.

That's one side!

I recommend taking a rest period before switching up to work the other side. Your core especially will need it. You'll get more out of the other side by waiting for some recovery (at least a minute to 90 seconds) before hitting the opposing movements.

It's going to look exactly the same only with sides reversed. I just shifted the bench over to the other side because I have a wall in the way. If you have a wall, you can just move the dumbbell to the other side of the bench and leave the set-up as-is. You'll just be facing the other way.

Get the dumbbell onto your lap, then reach up and grab the cable handle.

Scoot your butt forward off the bench, and then lie with your shoulders on the bench.

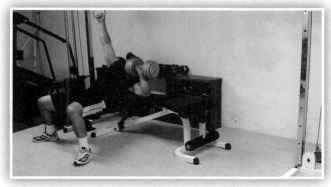

Press up with your left and pull down with your right.

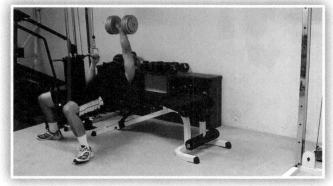

Repeat for 5 or 6 reps.

All done!

I would suggest two sets on each side and you'll be pretty well all done with your upper body training for the day. It's not only a great timesaver but KILLER core training as well.

If you've never really felt your deep abdominal muscles after training THIS exercise is going to change that!

RACK-RAIL LEG RAISES

T his one is a variation on the classic "leg raise" exercise. The key difference here lies in WHERE you're doing the exercise.

It's not a hanging version—it's actually a fair bit harder than that!

With this version, you're going to be supporting yourself on the safety rails of the power rack. It almost looks a bit like the Iron Cross position a gymnast does on the rings.

So first, set the safety rails on the rack to about the level of the bottom of your rib cage. You can adjust the height any time. I like to set the height so that I can set my hands on the rails while in a standing position, and then bend my knees to get my feet off the ground. I find this to be easier than trying to jump up in order to have straight legs at the bottom.

The arms should be about 45 degrees at the shoulder.

Set your hands on the rails and hold on! Bend your knees and get your feet off the ground. You will instantly feel big-time tension in the abs and torso because of how you're supporting your body in this position.

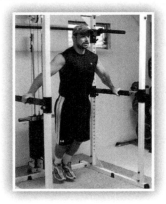

Now we add in the leg raise:

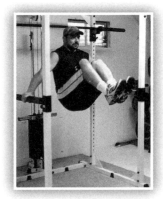

I like to start with the straight(ish) leg raise, then as I get tired, switch to the knee raise in order to keep going.

This one is BRUTAL because not only are you raising the legs (which involves the abs in a movement capacity), you're also involving the abs very intensely in a supporting capacity.

Give this one a try in your next ab-training session (do it first, before any other abdominal exercises—trust me on this--you probably won't need to do any more abs after a few sets of this).

RESTING GOBLET SQUATS

The Dumbbell Goblet Squat is an excellent leg, core and even upper body exercise. To perform that exercise, you simply hold a single dumbbell in a vertical position with your hands cradled under the plates, like you're holding a big goblet in your hands. Hold that at chest level, then squat.

This version of the Goblet Squat adds a small twist to the exercise...literally. At the bottom of each rep, you're going to rest the dumbbell, on end, on first your right thigh, then stand up, then down and rest it on your left thigh.

This will hit the oblique muscles and transverse abdominus to a greater degree than with the straight up and down version. The twist is very small, but because the tension is shifted over as you start out of the bottom, you'll get some excellent core work, especially when you start using heavier dumbbells.

So first, get a moderate weight dumbbell. I'm using a 105 lb dumbbell because I've done this exercise before. Hold it with both hands.

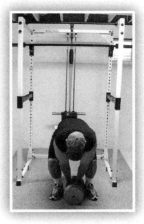

Squat down and rest it on your thigh, then get your palms under the top set of plates. This is the easiest way to get a heavier dumbbell into position for the exercise.

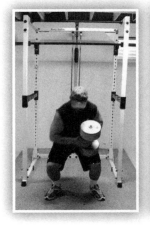 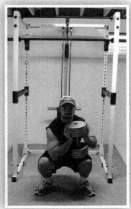

Now stand up.

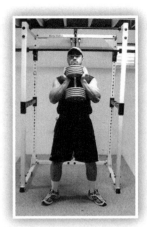

Now squat down, resting part of the dumbbell on your left thigh. Take tension completely off the hips and core at the bottom; we actually WANT to start from a dead stop here to develop power.

The other benefit is that you can reset your lower back arch and hips on every rep to make sure you're in the best squatting position. Hold your breath when you begin the push back up to stabilize the torso.

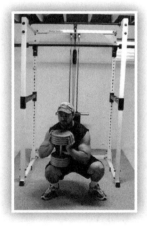

Stand up.

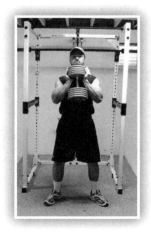

Squat again and rest it on the right thigh. As you can see, it's not completely on the thigh, just the outer half of the dumbbell plate. We don't want to twist much at all; it's a very subtle movement, basically shifting the weight to one side rather than fully twisting. This weight shift is what activates the oblique muscles.

Here's a side view of the goblet squat position.

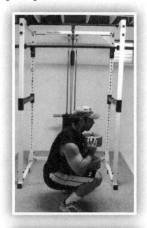

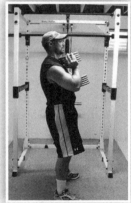

This Goblet Squat has a lot of benefits and adjusting it in this fashion can increase the core workload very effectively without excessive twisting because, as I mentioned above, it's really about shifting the weight a bit rather than really twisting very much.

The Goblet Squat in general is a great way to learn proper squat form. Having the weight in front of your body forces you to sit back in order to compensate for it and counterbalance against it, which is what you should do with a squat anyway.

SWISS BALL ROLL-UPS

This one of my favorite lower abdominal exercises (there is some debate as to whether you can actually focus tension on one area of the abdominal wall or not. My opinion is that you can't specifically ACTIVATE only one section or area of a muscle but you can, by using different body positions and leverages, work specific areas with more focused effort).

So even though you're not totally isolating the lower abs, you're putting your body in a position where the lower part of the abdominal wall is responsible for more of the movement.

Anyway, this exercise is excellent because it impacts the lower abdominal area without putting a lot of torque on the lower back, which exercises such as leg raises tend to do.

To do this one, you'll need a Swiss ball and a decline bench.

Move the bench in front of something solid like a rack, machine, or solid vertical post. The high end of the bench should be against the solid object, since this is what you'll be holding on to during the exercise. The higher the angle of the bench, the harder this exercise is, so when you first try it start with a fairly low angle on the bench.

Place the ball on the bench, about halfway up. Exactly where you set the ball to start will depend on the bench length and your height. This will take a little trial and error in order to get comfortable. When you see how the exercise is done, it will give you a better idea of where you need to place it to start.

Lay facedown on top of the ball, resting your elbows on the kneepads at the top of the bench and grab the solid object in front of it. The ball should be under your thighs, your arms slightly bent and body straight. The point in time when you set your thighs on the ball and take your feet off the ground is when you'll be the most unstable during this exercise. Hang on tightly and set your thighs fairly wide on the ball the first time you do it. This will give you more control over the ball until you get used to the movement.

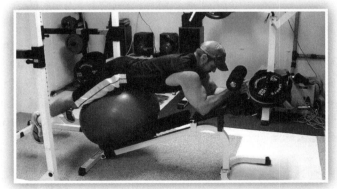

Now for the work.

Using abdominal power, roll the ball up the decline bench, bringing your knees up into your chest. The ball will roll down your legs as you pull your knees up and in. This results in an extremely strong contraction in the lower abs and the abs in general, so squeeze very hard and hold it for a few seconds. You can also bend at the shoulders while doing this exercise. Remember, you're going to be very unstable on the ball while you're doing this exercise so hold on tight! If the ball rolls off the bench, just put it back on and start again.

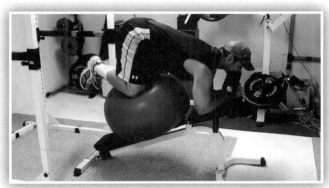

That's the exercise! I know you'll get some strange looks when you do this one but I also know that you'll see those same people trying that exercise when you come back the next day.

BACK

CORNER RACK PULL-UPS

If you want wider latissimus dorsii (lats), have I got an exercise for you! This one will blow them up like no other type of pull-up I've found. The secret to this one lies in WHERE you do the pull-up.

But I'm not very good at keeping secrets so here it is:

You do the pull-ups in the CORNER of the power rack!

I know it's hard to contain yourself at this point, but try to keep it together! Once I explain HOW to do pull-ups in the corner of the rack and WHY this corner pull-up works so well, you'll be itching to get to the gym and try it.

To really properly explain why it works so well, you first need to know how to do it so you can visualize how it works.

Now, to do this exercise, you're going to need a power rack. And that's pretty much it. Technically, you should also be able to do at least 6 to 8 reps of regular pull-ups in order to perform this exercise. But even if you CAN'T do that, I'm also going to show you a way to spot yourself so you CAN perform this exercise and get just as much out of it as someone who can.

So even if you can't do full pull-ups right now, keep reading!

First, stand facing the corner of the rack. Now reach up with your left hand and grip the top crossbar with a PALM-FACING-AWAY grip (a.k.a. reverse grip) about 18 inches from the corner. Now reach up with your right hand and grip the side top beam with the same grip at the same relative distance from the corner as your left hand. You want to be sure to keep your grip even on the beams. Definitely experiment with grip width to best match your arm span when performing this exercise.

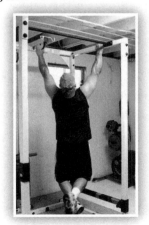

Now you're ready to pull!

Bend your knees to get your feet off the ground. You'll immediately notice the tension in your lats while in that bottom position. Perform a regular pull-up movement, bringing your body up as high as possible.

Here's the BIG trick: as you pull yourself up, try to consciously PUSH OUTWARD against the crossbeams of the rack. This outward pushing combined with the pulling up puts HUGE tension on the extreme outer fibers of the lats.

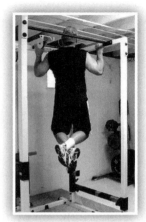

Pull yourself up as high as possible, then lower yourself SLOWLY and under complete control. The negative during this exercise is VERY intense and the stretch it puts on your lats is phenomenal!

As you get near the bottom, straighten your arms completely to maximize the stretch on the lats. Be sure to keep tension in the shoulders, though. Even though your arms are straight, you want your body to still be supported by muscle tension in the latissimus muscles and not the tendons and ligaments of your shoulder joints.

Now pull up again, remembering to push outwards against the crossbeams.

Keep going until you can't do any more reps. It is a tough exercise and an eye-opener even for people who can do a lot of pull-ups!

So how do you do this exercise if you can't do many (or any) pull-ups? Self-spotting with your feet.

When you're in the rack, you can either set the safety rail or the racking pin (the hook that you rack the weight onto) at about two feet or so off the ground. The exact height will depend on how tall your rack is and how tall you are. Basically, you're going to be using it as a step. As you do the pull-up, set your foot on that pin/rail and use your legs to help you.

It's important to give yourself only as much help as you need to complete the rep you're doing, NOT so much that you're just standing up and down and going through the motions. You want to keep strong tension on the lats to get the most out of this exercise.

CORNER PULL-UPS-SELF SPOTTING

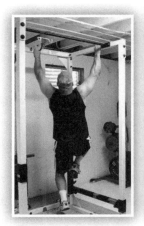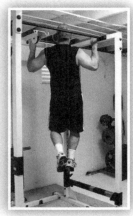

This technique is good not only for those who need help right off the bat, but also for doing forced reps when you CAN do full reps on your own. When you can't perform another full rep on your own, set your foot on the pin/rail and keep going!

You can also perform this exercise using a palms-facing-in grip (supinated), but I've found it to be less effective in terms of hitting the outer lats than the palms-facing-out version, because you don't get the same outward-pushing tension.

CORNER PULL-UPS SUPINATED GRIP

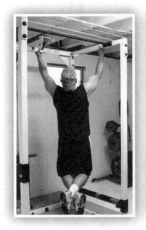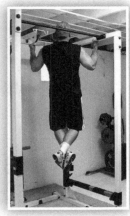

CROSS-BAND PULL-UPS

The wide-grip pull-up is a classic back exercise; everybody has seen this and knows basically how to do it, so I won't go into great detail about those.

This variation, done with two training bands, is going to work the lateral fibers of the lats even HARDER than the normal version.

To do this one, you'll need a couple of training bands:

http://www.fitstep.com/goto/ironwoody-bands.htm

I also recommend doing these on the chin-up bar found on most power racks (or on a Smith machine with the bar set to the highest position). The reason is you'll need something at the ends of the bar to hitch the bands onto to make this exercise work.

First, hitch the bands to the top/side cross beam of the rack, right next the chin-up bar (mine are in front of the bar). Put your right wrist through the loop of the left band.

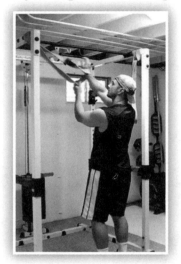

Next, put your left wrist through the loop of the right band.

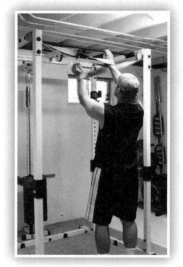

Now, reach wide to the ends of the bar, stretching both bands so that they cross in front of you. Your grip should be wide enough that the bands get some decent stretch. You're going to keep this grip through the entire set.

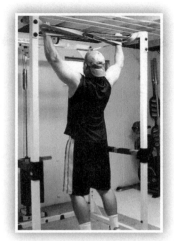

In this exercise, you're not going to be actively pulling against the bands; they're simply going to be supplying constant lateral tension against the wrists as you do the exercise. This tension activates the lateral fibers of the lats, which are responsible for upper lat width.

If lat width is something you want more of, this exercise is going to do it for you.

It also gives you nearly continuous tension on the lats, even at the bottom of the movement, where they would normally get a bit of a break. No break here.

Once you have a grip on the bar, lift your feet off the ground (or bench, if you're standing on one to get into position).

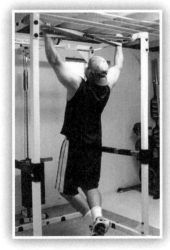

You'll be feeling the tension on your lats even before you start. Now when you start the pull, you'll REALLY feel it in the outer lat fibers. Pull all the way up, as high as you can.

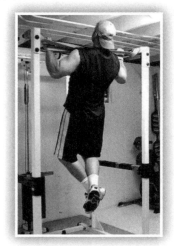

Go for as many reps as you can with good form.

If you'd like to extend the set, you can set the safety rails in the rack to a couple of feet off the ground and set your feet on those rails. This removes some of your bodyweight and you can adjust resistance using leg power.

This also allows you to get more reps and forces a full range of motion on those reps.

By the time you're done, your lats will be on fire and pumped up beyond recognition; I can promise you that.

DECLINE LYING PULLDOWNS

I f you have a hard time feeling your back working or if you're interesting really getting wider lats, you're going to LOVE this exercise. It'll trash your lats like crazy!

It's a very simple concept: basically, you're going to be doing a pulldown movement, but instead of sitting in a pulldown machine and doing them with a vertical body position, you're going to be lying on a decline bench and pulling the low cable forward and up.

Hard to explain with just words, but the pictures will show it well.

This one combines the benefits of the pulldown movement with the stretch of the pullover movement for the lats. It's a great overall latissimus developer.

First, set the decline bench in front of the low pulley. I like the V-bar for this one but you could instead use a straight bar handle.

Make sure the bench is a few feet away from the cable so that you have to reach fully overhead to grab the handle (this allows you to get the stretch on every rep).

Lie back on the bench, reach overhead and grab the handle.

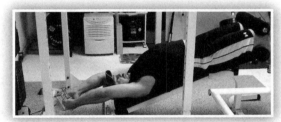

Now, using a standard pulldown movement, pull the handle towards your abdomen.

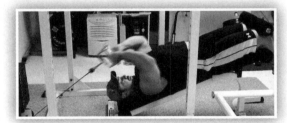

Pull the handle as far as you can (generally until it reaches about mid-chest level). Squeeze hard, then return it slowly back to the start position.

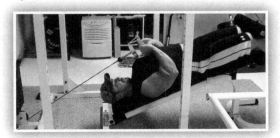

Let the weight pull a good stretch in your lats at the top. You'll find as you're doing the movement, this cable position and your body angle keep the tension on the lats from start to finish. You don't need a heavy weight to rip up the lats on this exercise.

Go for at least 8 to 12 reps per set on this exercise; it's a feel-based exercise rather than a power-based exercise.

ELEVATED RENEGADE ROWS

T he Renegade Row is a nice back and core exercise that's very straightforward to perform. It's like combining a plank with a one-arm dumbbell or kettlebell row movement. You hold yourself up on one arm while rowing the weight upward with the other.

The single-side resistance puts tremendous tension on the core while you're getting some good back work. This version of the Renegade Row has one big difference: instead of having your feet on the floor, they'll be up on a flat bench so that your body angle is on a decline. This changes where the exercise hits your core (more in the lower aspect, with a lot of tension going through the adductor muscles). It also changes the angle on your back training a bit, too.

To do this one, you'll need a flat bench and two dumbbells. Use weights that you can very easily do rows with. I'm just using 65 lb dumbbells here and I can row about three times that much for one-arm dumbbell rows. It's your core that's going to determine how much weight you can use for this one.

Set your hands on the dumbbells, then set your toes on the bench with your feet wide. You want to form a triangle with your base of support, since it'll be two feet and one hand. Start with your body in a straight plank position.

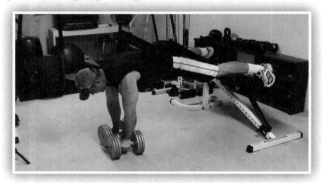

Now row up one dumbbell. You'll have to angle your body a bit to do the row and you'll have to tighten the adductors and core strongly to maintain your body position on the bench.

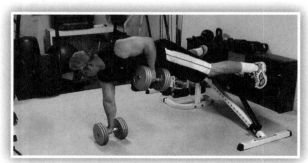

Set the dumbbell back on the floor.

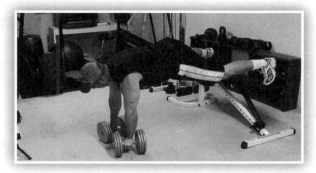

Row with the other arm.

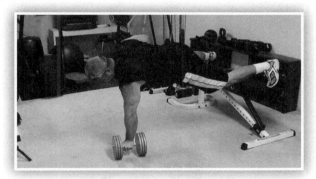

Make sure you keep the supporting arm locked out straight and keep your body as straight as possible.

It's a tough exercise for the core, even though the rowing part is not probably going to be all that challenging using the lighter weight.

Definitely a nice "change of pace" exercise that will hit your body in a unique fashion!

HAND-OVER-HAND CHIN-UPS

This one is a GREAT chin-up exercise that will blow your lats and your biceps up like crazy!

To perform it, you should be able to do at least eight to ten regular chin-ups. It's a tough exercise and requires some basic chinning strength to perform.

For this one, you'll just need a chin-up bar. I'm using the one that goes across the frame of my power rack and that works just fine.

So first, stand perpendicularly under the bar, so that you are facing the side. (NOT like you normally would directly under the bar).

Grip the bar like a baseball bat (staggered grip).

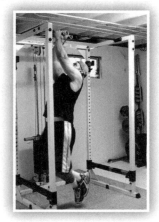

Now pull yourself up to one side of the bar. The side you'll want to pull to is the same as the hand that is forward on the bar. Basically, if your left hand is forward, pull up on the left side of the bar.

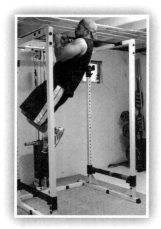

Now lower yourself down PART WAY...NOT the whole way. You should have some bend in your elbows. At this point, move your forward hand over behind the other hand (hence the hand-over-hand name!).

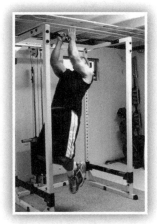

The key here is to be sure you've got a bend in the elbows and tension on the lats, because when you take one hand off, you're putting your entire bodyweight (just for a moment) on the one lat. VERY big-time tension here.

Once you've placed the hand, pull yourself up to the OTHER side.

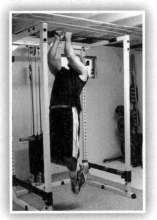

Lower yourself down, step your hand backward on the bar again.

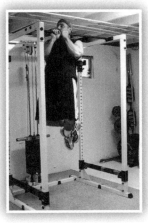

Now pull up to the other side again.

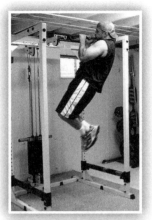

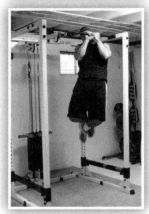

Continue along the bar until you run out of bar, then go back the way you came, moving your hands forward this time.

Keep going forward and backward along the bar until you can't do any more reps.

It's a BRUTAL back exercise that makes regular chin-ups look like nothing. By the time you're done, your entire back and your biceps will be so swollen and full of blood, you won't believe it. The continuous tension and bodyweight combination really makes for a potent back attack!

NECK-FOCUSED WEIGHTED DIPS

This exercise is not your normal weighted dip. Instead of having the dip belt around your waist, like you normally would, you're going to have the belt around the back of your head and neck.

This means while you're doing the dip, you're also getting some isometric neck work as well.

The first thing to note here is that you should start VERY light the first time you try it. It's perfectly safe to work the neck in an isometric fashion like this, you just want to be sure never to overload and strain those muscles.

So start light and work your way up gradually. I do a lot of heavy posterior chain training, which is why I'm using 45 pounds to start with in the demo, then increased to 90 pounds. This level of weight is fine for me because I'm advanced. Even if you are advanced like this, too, I would recommend starting lighter and moving up in small increments.

Set the belt around the back of your head and neck, and then get into position on the dip bars.

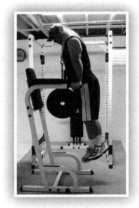

Lower down to the bottom of a dip. Having the weight around your head means your body will tilt forward as you come to the bottom, making it more of a chest dip at the bottom and a triceps dip at the top.

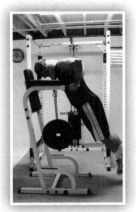

Keep your neck muscles tight and solid through the duration of the set—no relaxation. This is also going to work the upper trapezius fibers as well.

Obviously, you'll need to be strong enough to be able to actually DO weighted dips in the first place before attempting this exercise.

ONE ARM CABLE BACK EXTENSIONS

This is an exercise that actually surprised me with how good it felt, and I actually made it a staple of my training after that!

It's not a heavy exercise, it's a back extension done with lateral-pulling resistance from the cable, which immediately activates the lateral stabilizing muscles of the lower back and spine.

Here's the good part: it involves NO twisting of the spine even though it works the lateral and rotational-stabilizing muscles. The uneven resistance on the body is what forces that activation by PREVENTING rotation and twisting.

It's an extremely effective exercise that really hit my lower back and mid-back in a way I had never experienced before and is DEFINITELY worth trying out. Do just a few sets at the end of each workout, aiming for about six to eight reps per set.

To do this, you'll need a low pulley and a moveable hyper bench (a 45 degree one will work the best).

Center the bench between two pulleys (or if you just have one, set it about four or five feet away) and a little back from being in-line. You'll see why it needs to be a bit back when you see the exercise in action.

Go to the left pulley and grab it with your left hand. Use a light weight for this, only a couple of notches on the cable stack, especially the first time you do it. As I mentioned, it's NOT a heavy exercise; it directs unilateral resistance through your torso, forcing the small stabilizing muscles of the spine to activate to counter that torque.

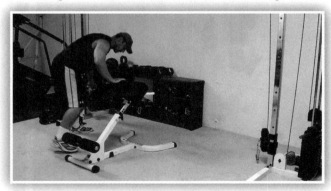

Get in position on the hyper bench as you normally would for a back extension, but holding your left arm (and the cable) directly out to the side, with your right arm behind your back.

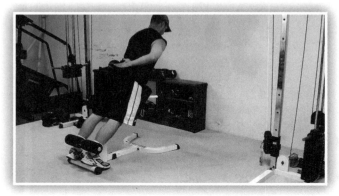

Now lower to the bottom of the extension. Keep that arm STRAIGHT out to the side. The only function of the weight here is to provide lateral-pulling tension on the body.

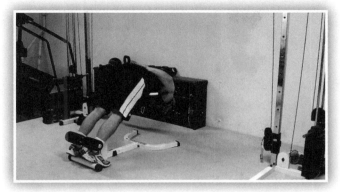

Perform these very deliberately and with tight form. Because the pull is coming from the left, you'll need to push with your left foot a bit harder to maintain balance.

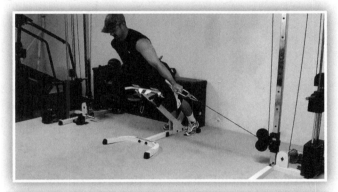

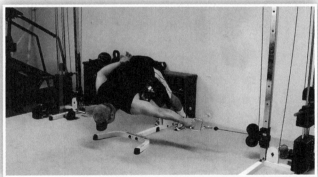

Once you've performed your reps on one side, switch to the other.

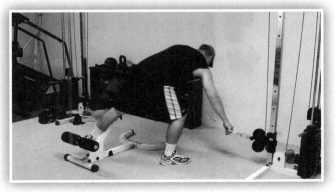

This gives you a good view of how the cable is held. Here you can see exactly why the bench needs to be a bit back from the line of the cable.

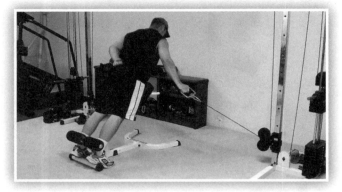

Go down into the extension, keeping that arm straight out to the side.

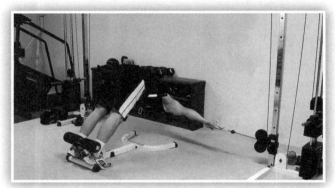

That's the exercise! It's performed almost exactly like a normal back extension; the lateral pulling tension is going to really hit those small stabilizer muscles of the lower back and spine and help you develop much better spinal strength and stability, while also working the bigger spinal erector muscles.

SEATED DEADLIFTS

S o I know you're already thinking, how in the heck can a person do deadlifts in a seated position? Easy! You just need something to sit on.

But first, what's the point of doing deadlifts in a seated position? Well, this is an especially useful exercise when you want to directly train the lower back for the top half of the deadlift.

This seated version takes the legs ALMOST completely out of the exercise (notice the almost—you need your legs for stability and isometric push), basically leaving your lower back to foot the bill when bringing the barbell up from the floor.

I use this one when I want to hit a heavy lower back movement but my legs are too trashed or I'm feeling tired and not up for full deadlifts. Like I mentioned, it's great for targeting the upper half of the deadlift, especially if you don't have a rack to work with. It directly works the lower back.

You'll need a sturdy bench for this exercise.

Load a barbell and set it just in front of the end of the bench, then sit on the very END of the bench. Start with moderate weight, but feel free to work up to some heavy weights as you're able to.

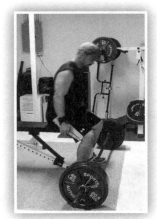

Now here's the trick. Step over the bar and roll it under your legs.

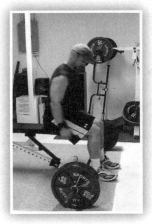

Lean forward and grab the bar with an overhand grip (or mixed or whatever your preference).

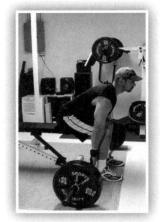

Now pull the bar up as you move into an upright seated position. As you begin the pull, tighten your entire core area. Solidify your abs and push your feet into the ground hard to brace your body.

Keep your lower back arched to protect your spine, and keep looking forward.

Here's the final position. Note the bar is coming up under your legs and under the bench.

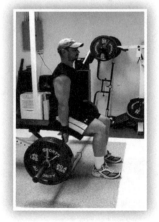

This exercise allows you to really focus on training the lower back effectively while not having overload your entire body with full-on deadlifts.

It's a good one! Don't be shy to use grip assistance when you get into the heavier weights. Personally, I use **1 Ton Hooks** for this purpose. They work like a charm for heavy gripping-intensive exercises. "1 Ton Hooks" are cast iron lifting hooks that are designed to allow you to hold extremely heavy without worrying about your grip strength. These hooks, in my opinion, should be in the arsenal of EVERY serious lifter and I highly recommend them. To put it in perspective, I've used these hooks to do partial deadlifts with more than 900 pounds and the hooks held up fine!

STIFF-LEGGED DEADLIFT PARTIALS
FOR BUILDING A THICKER BACK

As you might have gathered from reading some of the stuff in this book, I'm a big fan of repurposing exercises for targeting body parts other than the ones for which they were originally intended.

THAT is what this exercise is all about.

It's the top one-fourth of the Stiff-Legged Deadlift movement, done in the power rack but with a very important focus: instead of focusing on the hamstrings, you'll instead be pulling your back into a highly-contracted position, then doing the movement.

This is going to put the majority of the tension on those back muscles so that they get worked with about double the weight (or more) that they normally would with a rowing exercise.

The position at the shoulder blades resembles the top of the row (shoulders back) even though the arms stay straight. LOVE this one for building back thickness.

(I apologize for the frame on the pictures; the camera was a bit off-kilter).

You should be comfortable with the Stiff-Legged Deadlift exercise in general before doing this.

First, set the pins in the power rack to just above knee height and load the bar. I'm using 425 pounds in this one (which is about my 3 Rep Max for SLDL's).

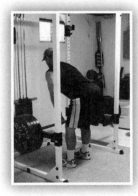

Now here's the important part: once you've gripped the bar, pull your chest towards the bar and pull your shoulders back, contracting all of your back muscles HARD and locking them there. You want to strive to keep this shoulders-back position through the entire movement.

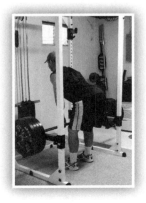

Now lift the bar off the rails. Keep your shoulders back and tight. You'll feel the tension of the weight trying to pull your shoulders forward; try to keep them back.

This exercise is also going to help your regular deadlift in that it'll help prevent your thoracic (upper) spine from curving forward. By building upper back strength, you can help minimize that curving.

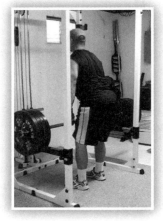

Come up to vertical, then lower the weight back down.

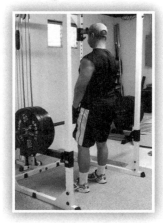

Set the bar fully on the rails and reset your back position. Then go again.

The first time you do this, you'll feel exactly how it's supposed to work. Pull your chest towards the bar, lock your shoulders back, and then lift. Keep the lower back arched the whole way, too.

This is GREAT for building thickness in the upper back. You could even say it's a great exercise for increasing your bench press; the thicker your back is, the shorter the range of motion the bar has to go in a bench press. A stronger back also helps better stabilize the bar during the movement, too.

SUITCASE-STYLE ONE ARM DEADLIFTS

The Suitcase-Style One Arm Deadlift is one of the most powerful, results-producing exercises you will NEVER see anybody in the gym do until you actually do it yourself! The reasons? First, it's NOT a common exercise, even though it's been around for many years. Second, it's a tough exercise to do! But as you know, the toughest exercises are always the most productive.

The Suitcase-Style One Arm Deadlift places extreme torque on the core and will help you develop an incredibly tight and powerful midsection. Basically, instead of using both arms and doing a barbell deadlift in front of your body as you normally would, you'll stand next to the barbell and pick it up with one arm.

Imagine reaching down and picking up a suitcase sitting beside you. That's the Suitcase-Style One Arm Deadlift but, of course, using a heavy barbell!

First, if you're doing this exercise off the floor, load a barbell with a 45-lb plate on each end. To lift this amount of weight, you should be able to deadlift at least 250 to 275 pounds in a normal deadlift.

If you wish to use less weight for this exercise, set the safety rails in the power rack to just below knee height and load the bar with however much weight you want to use. The reason you'd want to use the rack is because if you're using smaller plates, the bar will start too low to the ground and you'll need to lean over too far to the side to pick it up.

Stand beside the barbell and reach down and grasp it with one hand. When you do the One-Arm Deadlift, you should grip the bar slightly off-center. Your thumb and index finger grip should be about a centimeter (about a half inch or so) from the edge of the center grip surface. This uneven grip will prevent the bar being lifted unevenly and tilting as you are lifting.

The reason for this is that when you grip the bar with one hand, your thumb and forefinger grip area becomes the main pivot point. If that main pivot point is not close to the real center of the bar, the bar will tilt when you pick it up. By sliding your hand down so that your thumb and forefinger grip area is closer to the real center, you will have a much easier time keeping the bar level.

Before you pick up the bar, make sure your shoulders are level and your entire core area is tightened up very strongly. Pick up the bar, focusing on keeping your shoulders level as much as possible. The weight of the bar on one side of the body will place an EXTREME stabilizing load on the other side of the body. You will be pushing HARD with the same side foot as you're pulling on the bar, e.g. if you're picking the bar up with your right arm, you'll be pushing hard with your right foot.

Keep your lower back tight and arched as you stand up.

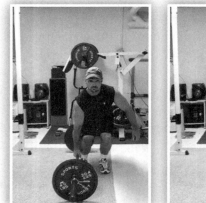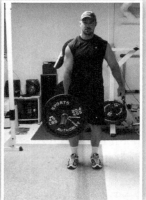

Come all the way up to the top position and hold for a few seconds, then lower the bar back down slowly.

Here's a side view of the exercise.

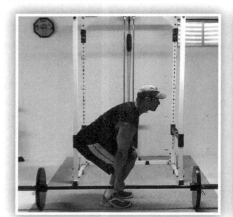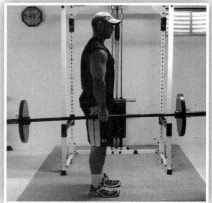

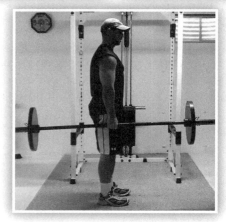

Gripping the barbell with one arm in this fashion is also VERY challenging to the grip. You'll need to hold on tightly in order to keep your grip on the bar.

Set the bar on the floor between reps and relax the core. Re-tighten everything before starting the next rep.

This exercise should only be done with low reps, e.g. three to five reps per set. Any more than that and the stabilizing muscles of the abs will become fatigued and cause the torque to go into the lower back instead of the abs, where you want it.

You can go immediately to the other arm after doing all your reps on one side.

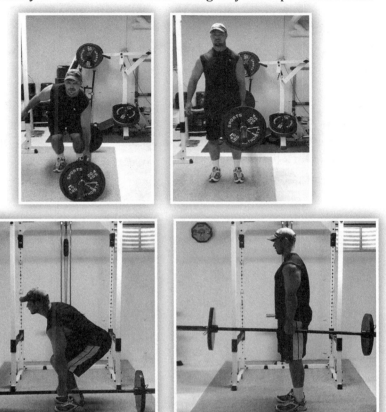

The first time you do this exercise, start with a conservative weight. It's deceptively tough, especially if you've not done a lot of movements that are weighted on only one side. The torque on your core will be a very new thing! The incredible tightness you'll feel all along the sides of your abs the next day will show you just how effective this exercise is.

If you're a strong deadlifter or find your grip strength limits the amount of weight or number of reps you can do, I would DEFINITELY recommend grip assistance in the form of either lifting straps or a product called "1

Ton Hooks." The grip assistance will allow you to use heavier weight and hold on to it longer. It will also prevent the bar from rolling out of your fingers as your grip fatigues.

I would recommend the hooks rather than the straps in all cases.

Give the Suitcase-Style One Arm Deadlift a try in your next back workout. I can promise you'll either be thanking me or cursing me for the next two days after you do it! Your entire core will be worked in a way it has NEVER been worked before.

WEIGHTED PULL-UPS ROWS

The pull-up row (a.k.a. Inverted Row) is a great bodyweight exercise for the back that you can do using just a low bar or rail.

THIS version adds resistance to the movement, increasing its value even more. And you can load some very substantial weight onto it!

You'll need a bar about three or four feet off the ground (this is where a rack comes in handy; you can set the height of the bar. A Smith machine bar will be perfect for this, too), a barbell and a bench or chair.

Set things up like in the picture below. The bar about four feet up (you'll have to play with bar height to get it right for the exercise), the bench a few feet away from the bar and a barbell on the floor in between. If you have a barbell pad, put that on, too, but a towel around the bar will work just as well.

Sit in the floor and slide your legs under the bar.

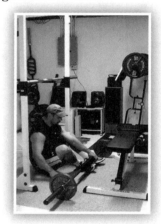

Set the bar on your waist, right about where the hipbones are (where you bend).

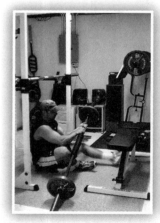 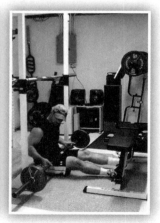

Now reach up and grab the bar in a pull-up grip (I'm using a close, underhand grip here).

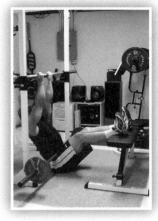

Put your feet up on the bench. Now you're ready to go!

Pull yourself up. As you can see, if you didn't have the bench, the bar would just roll down your legs—you need to maintain the bend in the waist to keep the bar cradled.

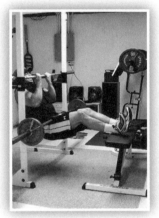

You can also perform this exercise with a wide, front grip. Use a lighter weight for this.

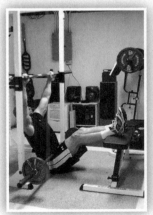 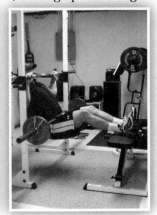

This weighted variation gives you a nice way to load the pull-up row exercise, though I've gotta be honest: in looking at these pictures, I should have used a lighter weight and leaned back more. These look more like pull-up positions more than they do a row.

You will definitely get some great back work out of it either way, though!

BICEPS

BARBELL INCLINE CURLS FOR MAXIMUM STRETCH

The stretch position of an exercise is one of the most productive positions you can put that target muscle in. It helps activate more muscle fibers by sending an emergency signal to the body and it can also help stretch out the fascia (the tough sheet of connective tissue surrounding the muscle that can restrict muscle growth), allowing more room for the muscles to grow.

This fascia-stretching aspect is best done after you've already performed other bicep exercises and filled the biceps with blood. It gives the fascia something to work against during the stretch (like squatting down in a pair of tight jeans just out of the laundry).

The best stretch exercise for the biceps is the incline curl, and it's generally done with dumbbells. THIS version, however, is going to use a barbell.

Now, you're probably wondering how you can use a barbell with the incline curl—won't the bar hit the bench? Absolutely it will, but we don't really care as much about what happens beyond the maximum stretch position. We're using only a very small portion of the range of motion to target a very specific position to put the biceps in.

The other question would be: why use a barbell at all when you CAN get a full range of motion with dumbbells? And the answer is that for maximum stretch (even beyond what you can get with a dumbbell), we actually WANT to lock the arms into position on the bar. With the arms locked in, it gives the muscles something to stretch against in addition to the stretch you get just with the incline position.

So by combining the inclined position with the locked-in-ness of the barbell, you actually get a greater stretch on the biceps than is possible with dumbbells in the exact same position.

And I'll tell you right up front: this degree of stretch is not comfortable. It won't injure you, but it's not comfortable. Also, if you DO have any bicep injuries or issues, you should skip this one because of the stretch-tension involved.

To do this, you'll either need a partner or a rack (you may also be able to do this one with a flat bench, too). If you have partner, you can just have them hand the bar to you and take it from you when you're done the set.

I've got the rack setup here, with an incline bench set with its high end in the rack. The barbell is set on the safety rails, which are just barely at arms-length when I get into position on the bench. If you want to try this with a flat bench, the bar will be resting on a bench set behind you.

Use a light weight for this; it's about the stretch, not how much weight you can load onto the bar. You don't need a whole lot of weight to get that stretch. I've only got 10 pounds on each side of the bar and that was plenty.

You'll also notice that I'm not sitting on the bench as I would normally. I've got my feet on the seat and my upper back is over the end of the bench. During the exercise itself, I'm going to basically be laying back over that top end of the bench while forcing the chest out and allowing the shoulders to stretch back more, which puts an even greater stretch on the biceps.

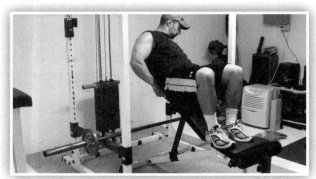

Lean down on one side and grasp the bar, then lean down to the other side to get the other hand on the bar. This is how you'll have to do it since you want to be sure those rack rails are not so high that you can just reach back and grab the bar, because that'll mean the bar will rest on the rails during the stretch part of the exercise itself. And that will basically defeat the whole purpose of this setup!

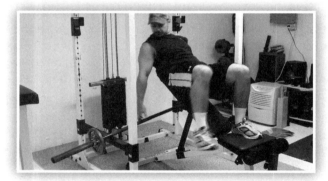

Once you've picked up the bar, lay back against the top end of the bench, letting the weight pull your shoulders and arms back and down. You'll instantly notice a MASSIVE stretch on the biceps. Hold that for at least five seconds.

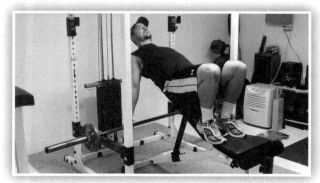

Now, curl up until the bar hits the back of the bench. You can either just touch the bench or you can do a static hold, pushing the bar against the bench for a few seconds.

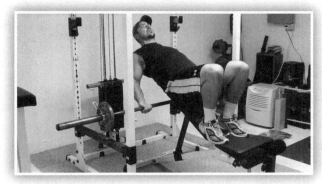

Lower back into the stretch slowly and hold again before repeating the sequence.

Aim for 4 to 6 stretch reps on this one. That stretch position is basically the maximum anatomical stretch you can put on the biceps, and it's going to be intense.

When you're done, because the rails should be set just below the bottom position, just unroll your grip on the bar and set it back down on the rails to finish. If you have a partner, they can just take the bar from you.

As I mentioned above, this is a great exercise to do AFTER you've already done another bicep exercise to fill the muscle with blood, giving you something to stretch the fascia against. Barbell or dumbbells curls are a good example of this.

BENCH STOP BARBELL CURLS

The Barbell Curl is an exercise that just lends itself to poor form; swinging out of the bottom to try and heave more weight up is the most common problem you'll see.

THIS technique is going to put a complete stop to that and all you need is a vertical bench.

It's also going to allow you to start the movement in a somewhat stretched position with ZERO momentum (you'll see why in a second), forcing ALL of the tension onto the biceps. It's a great form corrector.

So first, load up a barbell with a lighter weight than you think you'll need. Trust me on this, it's a humbling experience. I'm using a 95 pound barbell here and I can usually hit about ten to twelve reps with "normal" technique. With this technique, I think I could do just three or four reps.

Set the bar behind a vertical seat bench (like a shoulder press bench). The one I use is an adjustable bench that is set on a very steep incline.

Pick up the bar from the floor.

Now curl it to the top position and walk forward.

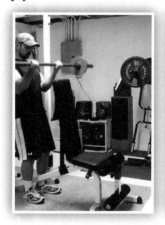 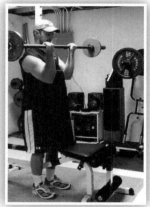

Press your chest up against the top of the bench and lower the barbell until it touches the front face of the bench. Relax your biceps to remove all elastic tension and make sure your arms are straight.

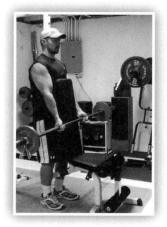

NOW begin the curl. You'll be amazed at how much tougher this is and how much tighter it forces the focus onto the biceps. Because you're starting with your arms a bit forward, you'll get no help from body position or momentum to start the movement.

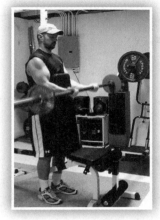

Come all the way up to the top and squeeze. It's important to note that your chest is just touching the bench, not resting or pushing on it and your arms are also not resting on top of the bench end. The bench is just there for the BOTTOM of the movement to stop the bar out in front of you, not to use for leverage.

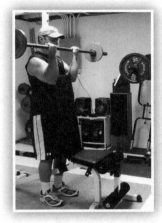

Do as many reps as you can with a full stop and bicep tension release at the bottom of each rep. When you're starting the lift out of the bottom, be sure to accelerate the bar with muscle power. Don't try to do a slow lift, really try and curl the bar fast. This position takes the momentum out of that and forces all the responsibility on the target muscles.

Once you've done your reps, finish at the top of a curl, then just step back and set the bar down.

Watch your step so you don't trip over the bench feet.

That's it! Simple to set up and perform, and really forces the right muscles to do the work.

BETTER INCLINE CURLS

The longer I train, the more I realize that even what you might normally think of as a basic exercise can be done MUCH more effectively with some very simple changes!

The Incline Dumbbell Curl is an example of this that I'd like to share with you here. The Incline Curl is one of THE most effective bicep-building exercises you can do. It puts a great stretch on the biceps at the bottom and can be a key exercise for major muscle growth.

And the standard way of setting up and performing the Incline Curl is just fine! There's nothing inherently wrong with lying back on an incline bench, letting your arms hang down beside you and curling the dumbbells up to the top position.

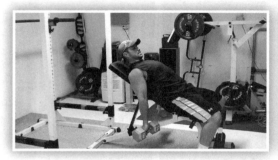 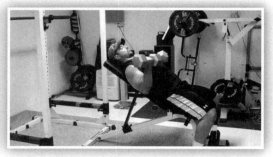

This "normal" way of doing the Incline Curl is very effective and time-tested. But you're NOT reading this because you want to settle for "normal" results!

So here's the simple technique for maximizing the results you get with the Incline Curl:

You're NOT going to sit on the seat of the incline bench as you normally would. First, pick up your dumbbells and straddle the incline bench.. Sit on the incline face of the bench, and set your FEET on the seat of the bench (knees bent).

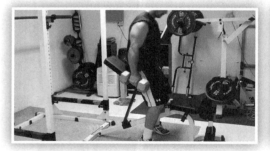 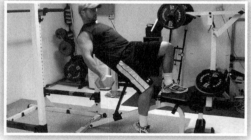

The top end of the bench should hit you just below the shoulder blades. Now arch your back over the top end of the bench. Turn your palms forward and keep them facing forward throughout the exercise for best results. In this bottom position, you should feel an increased stretch on the biceps beyond what you normally get with the Incline Curl.

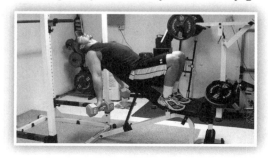

The reason this position results in an increased stretch on the biceps lies in the positioning of the chest and shoulders. The biceps attach in the shoulder joint. When you're in the standard position on the incline bench, your shoulders are braced on the bench and you can't fully open up your chest.

You do get a good stretch but it's not a MAXIMUM stretch, which is the key to massive results with this exercise!

When your shoulders are up and off the top end of the bench, the weight of the dumbbells pulls your shoulders back and down, opening up the chest and increasing the stretch on the biceps at the bottom.

Perform the exercise as you normally would an Incline Dumbbell Curl. Start the movement with a deliberate squeeze of the biceps, curl all the way up to the top, doing your best to keep the upper arms vertical (they may move up and forward a bit). Hold for a second at the top.

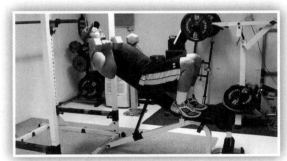

Now comes the payoff: on the way back down, DO NOT let your palms turn inwards. Keep them facing FORWARD all the way down to the bottom. This keeps full tension on the biceps all the way to the bottom, which is the most beneficial part of the exercise.

Lower the dumbbells under complete control. For an extra shot of tension, try to push your elbows forward as you lower the dumbbells. To do this, imagine as though you're trying to push a button with your bicep. It takes a bit of practice to get this feeling but it's definitely worth pursuing.

As you lower the dumbbells to the very bottom, let them pull and stretch your shoulders backwards and down, opening up the chest. This increased tension from the negative portion of the movement coupled with the greater stretch potential of your body position will give you an INCREDIBLE muscle-building stimulus. Take advantage of it and don't lose the stretch tension in your biceps!

Feel for that stretch, and then curl up again with a deliberate movement. When choosing weights for this exercise, start with weights that are lighter than you would normally use. When you apply stretch and tension to the biceps like this, it's a humbling experience in terms of the amount of weight you can use.

IN-SET SUPERSET-CURLS AND CHINS

This is a technique that I came up with that hits the biceps so effectively, you'll have trouble reaching up to scratch your nose without shaking. It's not really one exercise but a combination of two exercises that you've seen before.

The technique is called an In-Set Superset. Supersets are, in a nutshell, when you do two exercises in a row without taking any rest in between, e.g. bench press then immediately to flies. The purpose of this is to increase the stress on the target muscle. The In-Set Superset is slightly different than a regular Superset in that you alternate single reps of two different exercises WITHIN a set.

The example I used for triceps was combining Lying Triceps Extensions with Close Grip Bench Press. Basically, you do one rep of the extension, then immediately do one rep of the press, then extension, then press, etc., until you can't do any more extensions with the weight. You then finish by burning out on the presses until you can't do any more reps. This blows the triceps up like crazy!

Now, those exercises are very easy to transition between. You don't have to move anything or do anything to go from one to the other. And, they're different enough to stress the triceps from different angles.

For biceps, it's a bit trickier as there are not many exercises that are practical to switch between AND which are different enough to stress the bicep muscle fibers differently than just two types of curls.

THE SOLUTION: BARBELL CURLS AND CLOSE GRIP CHIN-UPS.

What we're going to do is alternate between doing a Barbell Curl (with an Olympic bar) then using that same barbell as a Chin-Up bar to do the chins on. The best place to perform this technique is in the power rack (a dip station can work if you don't have a rack available).

In the rack, set the racking hooks (the small hooks that you set the bar on for the start of an exercise) at about shoulder height. Set a bar on those hooks and load it with a weight you could curl for about ten to twelve reps. If you're using the dip station, set the bar on top of the dipping bars (everything else about the execution is exactly the same, you're just using the dip bars instead of the racking hooks to support the barbell).

Now stand directly in front of the bar (you should be inside the rack), step underneath it and turn around. You should be standing outside the rack facing in. The direction you face here is critical for the most natural execution of the two exercises.

Grip the bar with about a shoulder-width grip (we don't want a wide grip for the chins. Also, the closer grip is better for biceps activation on barbell curls).

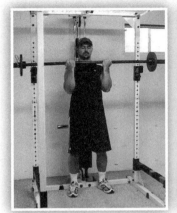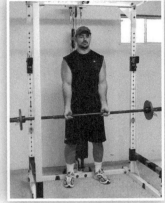

Lift the bar off the hooks and do a single barbell curl rep. Without removing your grip from the bar, set it in the hooks, lift your feet off the ground and pull them up into a cross-legged position in front of you. This position is necessary to keep your feet and knees from touching the ground during the chin.

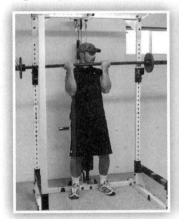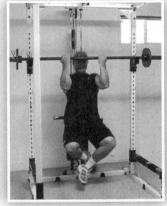

Lower yourself until your arms are straight, then pull yourself back up. Keep your torso vertical to maximize the tension on the biceps (this is one of the other benefits of the cross-legged position: holding your legs up in front of you keeps your torso vertical without even trying).

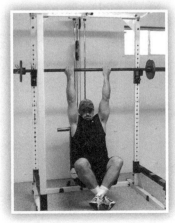

If you are unable to do chin-ups on your own, here's another great benefit of this exercise: you can keep your feet on the floor and use your legs to spot yourself as you come up! Just make sure that you're using as much bicep tension as possible and only using your legs enough to keep the movement going.

Setting your feet down and helping with your legs is also VERY valuable for stronger trainers as the biceps start to give out. You can really push your biceps hard by helping out with your legs as much as you need to.

At the top of the chin, set your feet back down on the floor, and without releasing your grip on the bar, immediately go into the next rep of the barbell curl.

Repeat this process until you can't do any more barbell curls in good form (it is permissible to use a bit of swinging to get a few "cheat" reps of the barbell curl to really push your biceps to the limit). When you're finished on barbell curls, you can either stop with your final chin-up rep or burn out with as many chin-ups as you can do.

At this point, I can promise that your biceps will be screaming! The emergency response from your body will send a rush of blood to your arms, resulting in one of the strongest pumps you'll ever experience. You will probably also find that your grip is being VERY strongly worked as well.

In addition, if you want to try this exercise from another angle and target brachialis development, do reverse-grip barbell curls alternated with reverse-grip chin-ups. You will need to lighten the weight to perform the reverse curls but the execution is exactly the same.

You can also alternate between sets of regular grip In-Set Supersets with sets of reverse-grip In-Set Supersets (resting in between Supersets, of course).

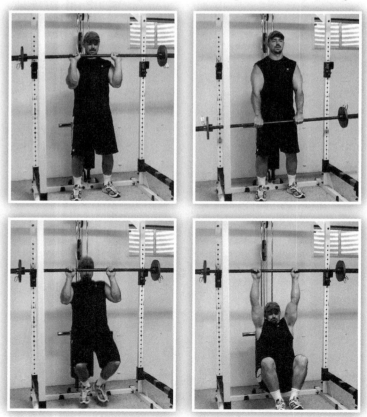

When you're done and you can't touch your nose because your biceps are so pumped up, you'll only have me to blame.

One of the main reasons this technique works so well is that you are going from a strong isolation exercise for the biceps (the Barbell Curl) immediately into a compound exercise for the biceps (when doing the chins, the back works with the biceps to complete the movement). Your back will help push your biceps to a whole new level!

Give this technique a try in your next biceps workout. As a person who has had to overcome poor genetics for biceps, I can tell you from experience, this exercise combination will make a HUGE difference in how your biceps respond to training.

KNEELING CABLE ROWS FOR BICEPS

T he biceps generally suffer from over-isolation...meaning most people who want to build their biceps tend to focus on the isolation exercises for the biceps, such as various forms of curls.

Now, there's nothing inherently wrong with doing curls; the only problem is that they won't build the biceps as much as compound exercises that involve biceps (such as chins and rows).

Involving the biceps in heavy, compound exercises is the REAL way to build biceps.

Now, what if you take a compound exercise (like the cable row) and adjust your body position and path of movement so that the biceps take more of the load?

That's what THIS exercise is all about. It's a cable row movement done in an "all fours" body position (which is actually "all threes" because one hand will be rowing).

It's a simple change in body position that still allows you to use fairly heavy weight with a compound movement while focusing on the biceps.

To do this one, you'll need a low pulley or seated cable row setup. Set a moderately heavy weight on the stack and attach a single cable handle.

Kneel in front of the stack and grab the handle.

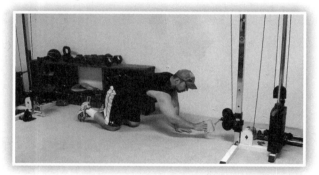

Now take a few steps back so your arm is fully stretched and the stack is off the bottom. This is the starting position. The hand on the ground will be bracing you from the weight pulling you forward, and this activates the core HARD when you perform the row as it becomes a push-pull type of cross-tension through the core.

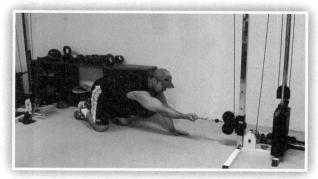

Row the handle in towards your body, keeping your torso down. Focus on pulling with the bicep and gripping the handle hard. As you row, try to bring the handle UP as you do it. This will help activate the bicep.

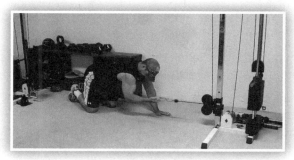

Row until your arm is fully flexed and squeeze the bicep hard.

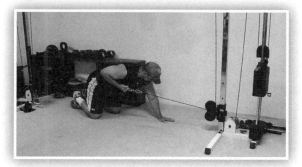

Lower and repeat for six to eight reps. Switch hands.

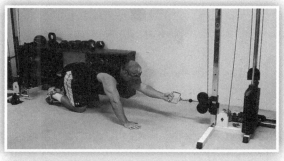

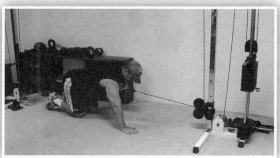

In this body position, your lats will be the secondary mover and the biceps will be the primary mover.

And, as I mentioned, your core is going to take a beating with the cross-tension from bracing yourself with your other hand. This is a nice added bonus.

NILSSON CURLS-THE BEST BICEP EXERCISE EVER...

I f you want to TRULY maximize your bicep mass, you're going to LOVE this exercise. It's one of my very favorites for building biceps.

The reason I named it after myself is that it basically summarizes what I'm all about: doing everything completely "backwards" and getting MUCH better results!

The Nilsson Curl looks almost exactly like a chin-up. In fact, another name I've called this exercise is the "Forearm-Braced Chin-Up," because what you'll be doing IS a chin-up. But, you'll be doing that chin-up with your forearms braced against another bar so that the VAST majority of the tension goes to your biceps instead of your back.

You'll need to be able to do probably six to ten or so regular full chin-ups before you can really use this exercise.

Think about it: imagine the kind of growth response you'll get from an exercise that puts the tension of almost your entire bodyweight directly onto your biceps.

That's the beauty of the exercise: it's a bodyweight exercise, which means increased muscle fiber activation.

To do this exercise, you'll need a rack or a chin-up bar that allows you to set another bar close underneath it. Alternatively, you can also use the metal ladder of playground apparatus (that works quite well, too).

Set the racking pins (where you would normally rack the bar on a squat, for instance) to the highest point you can.

Then, move the safety rails up to a point that is about eight to twelve inches below that (you can play with this height when you try the exercise to get the best dimensions for you).

Set a bar on the top racking pins and set another bar on the safety rails, pushed against the uprights. It's going to look like two rungs of a ladder.

In my setup, I load the top bar with weight plates to keep it from moving.

If you have a power rack that has pins that can slide in and out of the frame (I don't-mine are integrated right into the rack) you can also more easily get this set up by setting one safety rail in the top set of holes and the other safety rail in a set of holes below (making your own ladder, essentially). That's the easiest way to set this up and how I used to do it when I had access to a rack that I could do it with.

Now get in the rack and take a close, underhand grip on the top bar. Your forearms should be braced against the bottom bar, just above your elbows. Your arms should be straight.

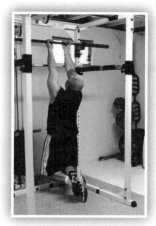

Now start doing a chin-up. As you pull yourself up, your forearms are pressed against the bottom bar, changing it to a biceps-oriented movement.

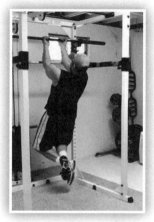

Pull yourself up all the way, then lower slowly.

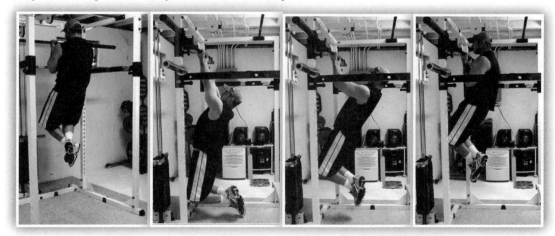

As you get stronger, you can also add weight by holding a dumbbell between your feet or wearing a dip belt. But that's VERY advanced. This exercise is just BRUTAL even with just your bodyweight.

Take this exercise for a spin on your next bicep workout. Do it FIRST in your bicep routine (trust me). You won't need to do pretty much anything else for bi's when you do three or four sets of this one.

ONE-ARM BARBELL CURLS

This is exactly what the name implies: a barbell curl with one arm. The concept is not hard to grasp but it's a GREAT exercise. Really fires up the biceps and the forearms.

Because not only do you have to do the curl, you have to balance a seven-foot-long Olympic bar in one hand as you're doing the exercise.

You can also do this exercise with a smaller bar (standard or EZ Curl) if you can't do a curl with the 45 pound O bar, so no worries there. You can also do it as a reverse curl.

Basically, grip the bar in the middle with your right hand. On the first rep, you'll see immediately how you need to adjust your grip in order to balance the bar. Shift your hand as you need to.

Because you're lifting with just one arm, it's going to throw your balance off a bit, so keep that in mind as you do the exercise. A little body lean is fine because of this.

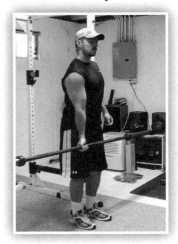

Then curl the barbell up to the top.

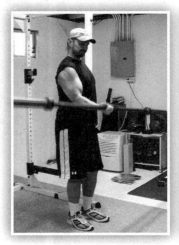
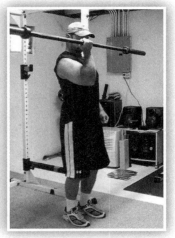

Do all your reps on one arm, then switch over to the other arm. You can also hold your other arm behind your back while doing this exercise.

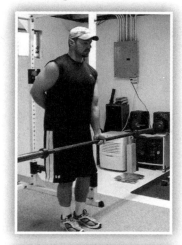

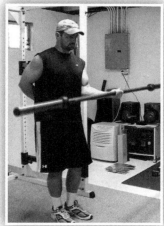

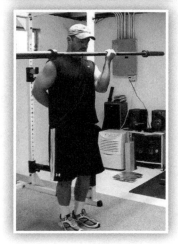

It's a pretty straightforward exercise but VERY challenging for the biceps, even with just the bar! Add weight slowly to this one since it's one-arm at a time.

That's the exercise! Simple to execute but VERY challenging.

SQUATTING CABLE CURLS

To maximally develop the bicep muscles, you need to apply tension to them in three distinct areas of their range of motion (if you are familiar with Steve Holman's "Positions of Flexion" training, you'll recognize these areas). Most bicep exercises work only one area at a time. The Squatting Cable Curl exercise you are about to learn works all three at once!

The first area is the stretch position. This position is worked in exercises that place the most tension on the muscle when it's stretched. This could be dumbbell flies for the chest or, for the biceps, incline curls. The body position of the incline curl (lying on an incline bench with your arms hanging straight down) puts a stretch on the biceps muscle at the start of the movement.

The second area is the midrange. This is just the middle of the movement. Exercises that have most of their tension placed in the middle of the movement work the midrange. For the biceps, this could be standing barbell or dumbbell curls. You'll notice that they are hardest when you are halfway through the movement (90 degree bend in the elbows).

The third area is the contracted position. Exercises that have the majority of their tension when the muscle is contracted, such as concentration curls for the biceps, work this third area.

Taken separately, each of these three areas contributes to full development of the muscle. For example, if you wanted to do a bicep routine based on this theory, you could do one set of incline curls, two sets of barbell curls, and then one set of concentration curls. This routine would ensure you are working all three tension-areas of the bicep.

But what if I told you there was an exercise you could do that would work all three of these areas at once? Each of the three movements I referred to above lose tension in the biceps at some point because of gravity and the positioning of the resistance. There is zero tension in the biceps at the bottom of the concentration curl. This factor decreases the effectiveness of the individual exercise.

The Squatting Cable Curl solves this tension-loss problem neatly and easily. First, I'll explain how to do it, then I'll tell you exactly how and why it works.

❧ ❧ ❧

To do this exercise, you will need a low pulley and a curl bar attachment (it can be the straight or cambered bar). There will be a link to pictures of the exercise at the end of the article.

Attach the bar to the low pulley and set a weight that is somewhat less than what you'd use for standing cable curls.

Squat all the way down (with your butt on your heels) and grasp the bar with a regular curl grip. Rest the top sections of your forearms on the tops of your knees. Take a small step back so that the plates on the weight stack are raised (you need to have tension at the bottom of the movement). You are going to be using your knees and then your elbows as the pivot points for this exercise.

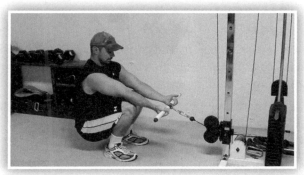

When your arms are straight in this position, you should notice that your biceps are getting stretched. The weight is pulling forward and down while your knees are bracing your arms. This exercise does require a bit of balance, especially when you are first getting used to it.

Start the curling movement, rolling your forearms up and over your knees. This rolling pivot point changes the angle of tension on the biceps all the way through the movement.

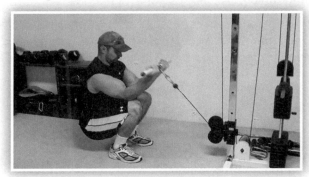

As your forearms roll up and over the top of your knees, the pivot point will then move to your elbows. This will again change the angle of tension of the exercise.

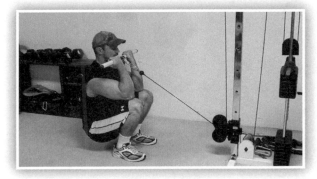

Continue the movement, curling the bar up as close to your face as possible. Squeeze the biceps hard at the top. You should feel an extremely powerful contraction at this point as your biceps have had tension on them for the entire movement. To increase the feeling of the contraction, you can lean your body back somewhat (as though you are about to roll backwards).

Now reverse the sequence, rolling your forearms down and over your knees again. Get a stretch at the bottom (with your arms completely straight and the weight pulling on the biceps), then repeat.

CR   CR   CR

The Squatting Cable Curl works by using the cable and your body parts and positioning to apply varying tension to the biceps. It applies tension to the biceps during all three areas of the movement: stretch, midrange and contracted positions.

At the very beginning of the movement, when your knees are pushing your elbows up and the weight is pulling your hands down, you are getting a strong biceps stretch. By applying tension to the biceps, i.e. curling the weight, you hit the stretch area.

As your forearms roll over your knees, the biomechanics of the movement change. You are now applying direct tension in the midrange of the exercise. The best part is, because you are rolling your forearms over your knees, the angle of pull is constantly changing. This means you are getting direct tension on the many different angles of the midrange area.

When you come to the point where your forearms roll completely off your knees and you begin pivoting from your elbows only, you are focusing on the contracted position. At this point, you can maximize the tension of the contraction by consciously squeezing the biceps hard and pulling the bar as close as you can to your face.

One of the bonuses of this exercise is the fact that your arms are braced against your legs throughout the movement. This effectively prevents any cheating due to body or arm movement. This bracing forces strict form, which makes the biceps do all the work in the exercise.

STRAIGHT BAR NEUTRAL-GRIP CHIN-UPS

The chin-up is one of the best exercises you can do for the back and biceps. This is a version that sets your hands in a neutral grip to change the focus of the exercise somewhat. It will allow you to keep your elbows in closer, working the lats a little differently, while the neutral grip targets the brachialis muscles more strongly (the muscles underneath the lower aspect of the biceps; when developed, these can help improve the peak of the biceps by pushing them up from below).

The trick is that instead of using handles designed for using that neutral (palms facing in) grip, you'll use the straight, normal chin-up bar.

You're going to hold the bar in a baseball bat grip, then pull yourself up to one side, pulling until your shoulder almost touches the bar.

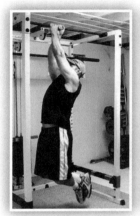 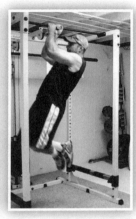 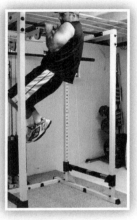

The movement is essentially the same as a regular chin-up; the main difference is the grip and how you pull yourself up in relation to the bar.

I like to do two reps on one side, set my feet down briefly before switching hands and pulling up to the other side. I find the most natural way to come up is the same side as the hand that's forward on the bar.

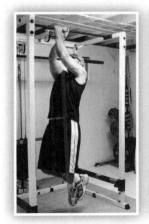 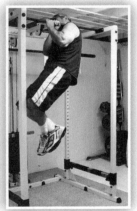

You'll notice this one really hits the brachialis muscles. That neutral grip coupled with the bodyweight resistance loads it nicely. Very good exercise for building arm size as well as hitting the back.

VERY CLOSE GRIP BARBELL ROWS

This is a back exercise that doubles as an upper arm exercise. I actually came up with this one as a way to do a compound exercise for the biceps that wasn't a pull-up.

So to do this, I focused on what made the barbell row hit the arms more; this is accomplished by moving the hands close together on the bar.

This results in greater elbow flexion during the movement (i.e.. the arms bend more), which means the upper arms take more of the brunt of the exercise.

This one DOES still hit the back (especially the teres major, rhomboids and posterior delts) because it is a rowing movement. But you'll really feel the focus on the upper arms, more the brachialis rather than the biceps because the hand position makes it work like a neutral-grip hammer curl.

Set up a barbell on the floor with a weight you'd find pretty easy to row with. I've got 135 pounds on the bar for this one. Grab it with an overhand grip with hands pressed right up against each other in the center of the bar.

Now, lift the bar to the bottom start position of the row, with the lower back arched and tight, knees bent, and core tight.

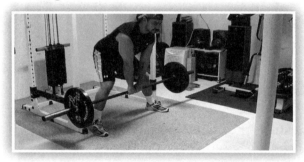

Row the bar up into your abdomen on whatever track feels best to you. Note the bend in the elbows as I get to the top; this puts a lot of tension on the upper arms when using a weight you'd have a hard time doing a reverse curl with.

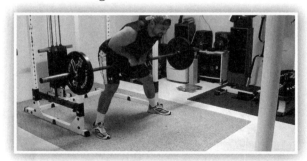

That's the movement: just row until your arms are toasted. It allows you to use your back muscles to push your upper arms to the limit.

I find exercises like this so useful for building arms because I find arms respond better to heavier-weight movements. For me, I'm actually not that strong in curls, yet I have 17 1/2" arms. I've seen guys who have only been training a few months who are able to curl more than I am.

It's the heavy rowing, pressing, chins and deadlifting movements that really build serious arm size. This is a great way to target a row for building arm size.

CALVES

BARBELL AND BENCH DONKEY CALF RAISES

If you train at home, you'll generally have a hard time finding calf exercises that are effective. Aside from standing calf raises with a dumbbell, there aren't a lot of easy options.

THIS is a good option; it'll allow you to do Donkey Calf Raises without a machine, without a rack and without a partner.

What you WILL need is a barbell and an adjustable incline bench (or a regular incline bench-adjustable is better). Ideally, you will also have a barbell pad...you'll see why it comes in handy.

First, set the incline so that the end of the bench is about at waist height. Set the barbell on the floor a few feet behind the bench and stand in front of the barbell. The barbell pad should be in the middle.

Squat down and grab the bar with an overhand grip, at a moderate-width. I was using middle fingers on the smooth rings.

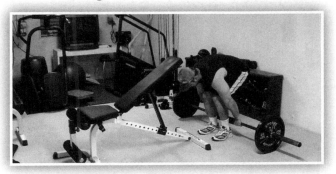

Now the interesting part: you're going to do a powerful behind-the-back barbell hack squat movement. And it should be powerful because you're going to pull the bar up as high as you can so you can rest it on your lower back.

You should be comfortable with deadlifting when doing this one. Your back won't be in a perfectly arched position, so it's something to be aware of when doing it. Personally, I had pretty much no back strain.

Keep pulling up until the bar is on your lower back, and then lean forward.

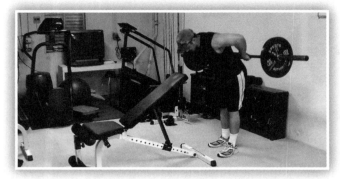

Step forward and set your toes on the feet of the bench, using that as your calf block. If your bench doesn't work like this, you may need to use a calf block and figure it out with your equipment.

Set your chest on the end of the bench, just below the pecs. The key here is you're using this bench end for

BALANCE, not for resting your whole bodyweight on. It's a balance point only.

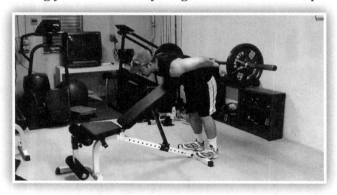

Stretch your calves by dropping your heels.

Then go up.

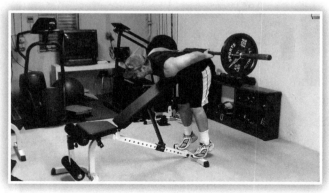

It's going to take some practice to get everything firing properly but it's actually a VERY good version of the donkey calf raise.

And the beauty of it is the very basic equipment needed to do it.

BARBELL END CALF RAISES

T he calf raise is not a glamorous exercise. I think we all know that. That doesn't mean you shouldn't train calves, though!

I have an exercise that is similar to seated calf raises that you can do with just a barbell (and a calf block, if you have one). This makes it VERY useful if you train at home and/or don't have access to a seated calf raise machine.

Set a plate or two on one end of the barbell (you can load the other end also to help keep it from rolling, but since you'll placing your leg outside the plate, it's not going to make the barbell end fly up).

Stand at the end of the bar, facing it. If the majority of the bar is to your left, put your RIGHT foot forward (I'll explain why this is important in a minute). Set it directly underneath the end of the barbell.

Reach down and pick up the barbell end and lift it onto your thigh, dropping down to one knee as you do so.

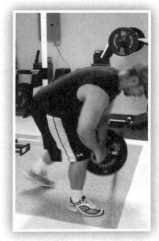

Here's what it looks like at the start position. Notice my knee is forward. Since my foot is flat on the floor, with no calf block, setting the knee forward increases the stretch at the ankle (which you can see in the picture), without needing a calf block.

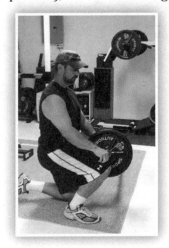

Now do a simple calf raise movement.

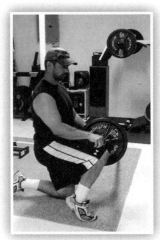

That's the exercise! Very simple and very easy to set up. When you're done with the reps, all you have to do is stand up and set the bar back on the floor.

Now, the reason you want the right foot forward is this: the big toe is the key to calf development.

By having your right foot forward when the resistance is to your left (and the bar is angled to your left) FORCES the tension of the calf raise to go through the big toe knuckle. There's no choice in the matter because that's how the bar moves.

So it forces you to move in the best path for calf development when you set the outside leg and foot forward. When you go the other side of the bar, you'll put your left foot forward and perform the same movement.

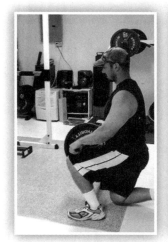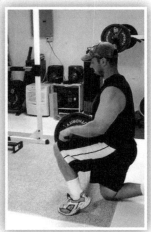

You can also do this with a calf block or foam wedge.

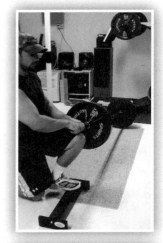

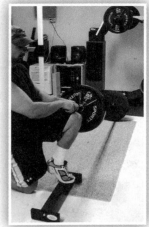

This is a great exercise for calf development using very simple equipment that is accessible even for home gym users with very little space.

CALF ROCK-UPS

T his is a bodyweight contracted position exercise for the calves that can be done anywhere at any time because it requires no equipment at all!

While it doesn't put a whole lot of resistance on the calves, the muscle contraction you can get with this one is AMAZING. It's an excellent finishing movement for the soleus muscles because it places them in the most contracted position that is anatomically possible.

It's a VERY simple exercise; all you need to do is squat down and hold onto something for balance. Squat down until your glutes are on your heels. Then come up on your toes, squeezing your calves as HARD as you can.

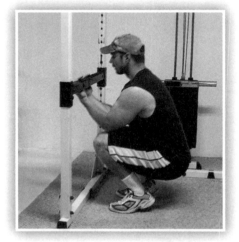

Hold that squeeze at the top and really dig to try to make your calves contract as hard as possible.

This has the other advantage of giving you a better mind-muscle connection with your calves, which will help you activate them more effectively in other exercises like seated calf raises.

Heck, give this exercise a try right now! Hold onto your computer desk for balance, squat down as far as you can then come up on your toes.

You WILL feel the exercise working on the very first rep!

And like I said above, this is better for a finishing movement (it'll help with shape and definition in the calves),

rather than something that will actually build a whole lot of mass in the calves.

Definitely a good tool for your training toolbox. It's a nice one for when you're travelling, too, because there is zero equipment required.

If you DO want to increase resistance, you can try it holding a weight plate or dumbbell on your knees.

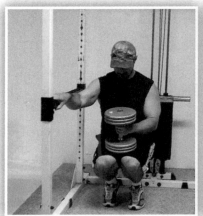 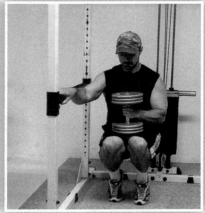

You can also use the Smith machine (I don't have a Smith machine to demo this on, unfortunately, but here's how I have done it in the past):

- Lower the bar to a point about a foot and a half off the ground. Use a foamy barbell pad if you have one or even a towel rolled around the bar.

- Place your feet slightly behind the bar, then tuck your knees under the bar so that the foamy pad is on the top of the thighs, just above the knees.

- You will be in an extreme squatting position with your heels slightly off the ground.

- Rise up onto the balls of your feet, squeezing hard.

- Keep tension in your thighs to prevent knee stress.

- Hang onto the bar to allow you to reset it at a moment's notice.

- These can be done one leg at a time, with your other leg behind as if you are in the bottom of the lunge position.

LENGTHWISE BARBELL DONKEY CALF RAISES

The Donkey Calf Raise is simply one of THE best exercises for developing the calves. The reason for this is the great stretch you can put on the calves at the bottom of every single rep.

Because the calf muscles (the gastrocnemius, to be specific) cross the knee joint, putting a stretch on the hamstrings also puts a greater stretch on the calves. So, bending over at the waist puts a greater stretch on your calves.

But here's the problem: when you don't have a donkey calf raise machine OR a partner to sit on your back (like they're riding a donkey, hence the name), how do you perform this exercise? Donkey machines are not

common in all gyms and if you're training at home, I have a feeling a donkey calf machine wasn't on your priority list of purchases (hopefully, a power rack was!).

One of the solutions I've come up with is using a dip belt to add resistance.

But it's not a perfect solution either. The weight doesn't sit in the best spot to get the most out of the exercise (it's more on the lower back than sitting on the hips, where you'd get the best effect). And, the stronger your calves are, the more plates you have to use. The more plates you have to use, the more awkward the exercise becomes and the wider you have to set your feet apart. It's not so bad when you're working with two or three plates. But I've gone as high as six plates and it gets VERY hard to perform the exercise effectively.

So here's my BETTER solution: a barbell along your back, set up in the power rack.

When you're doing the donkey calf raise, you want your legs to be pretty much straight and locked. Since we're not squatting down, the lower side rail needs to be a bit higher up than if you were doing the squat.

And because that one is a bit higher, the OTHER one needs to be a bit higher as well.

With this height, you're going to need a calf block to do the calf raise on. That's pretty much it. Play around with the height until you feel comfortable.

The thing to note is that when you're getting into position for the exercise, you SHOULD have to squat a little. You want to ensure you get a full stretch on the calves without the bar hitting the rail at the bottom of every rep. But playing around with bar height will give you the best feeling for where to set the rails.

Here's what it looks like: both ends of the barbell are loaded and I've got a barbell pad down near the hips for padding. A rolled-up towel will work as well.

Get your feet set on the calf block and get underneath the bar. Grab the bar near the other end, right by the rail. That's the pivot point, just like in the squat.

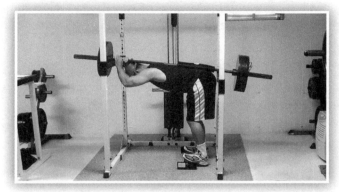

Now it's just a matter of coming up into a calf raise! At the bottom be VERY sure to get a deep stretch. Come up fully into the calf raise at the top.

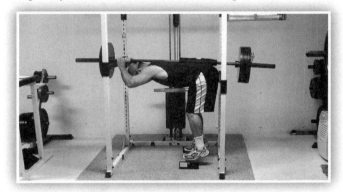

This exercise setup is every bit as good as any donkey calf raise machine I've ever used—better, in fact, because your body isn't locked into the movement. Because the end of the barbell moves freely, you're not locked into the exercise and your body can find its own groove.

Next time you're hitting calves in the gym, take a crack at this one. And never mind the strange looks you get from everybody else in the gym. You'll see THEM doing this exercise the next time you come to the gym.

ONE LEG BACK BARBELL CALF RAISES

I f you're training without much in the way of specific calf equipment (i.e. machines), it can be tough to really load the calves with enough resistance to make a difference.

But, in truth, if you've got some simple stuff like barbells, dumbbells and/or a power rack, you've got everything you need.

You may have seen barbell standing calf raises starting with your feet flat on the floor. This is a great exercise but obviously, it only hits HALF the range of motion of the calves. The stretch position is of great value in the calf raise exercise and needs to be hit as well.

How do you that with just a barbell? I'll show you!

First, load a barbell in the rack. You can use a pretty good amount of weight for this exercise because of the angle, even though you're working just one leg at a time. I've got 315 pounds on the bar here.

Set one foot back like you were about to set up for a split squat exercise. Don't set your feet directly in line, though. Make sure you have some horizontal separation so you've got a good base of support.

Note the position of my back leg. There's a stretch on that calf!

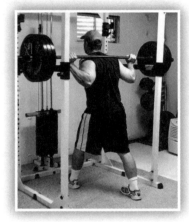

Now just do a single leg calf raise, pushing up on that back foot. Like I said, because of the angle, you can use a good amount of weight for this (and should!).

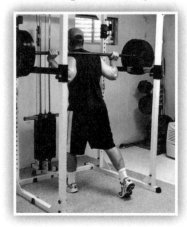

You'll be able to work that back calf through a full range of motion. The nice thing is, it's also a very practical position for increasing calf power in running; you're using the calves for FORWARD propulsion rather than just straight up and down as you do in a regular calf raise.

This is a very big benefit of this exercise, making it worthwhile even if you DO have standard calf equipment. Do your reps on one leg, then switch to the other.

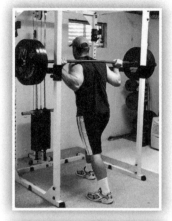

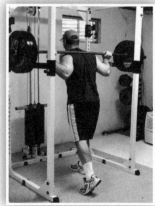

You're basically pushing off that back leg using just the calf to move forward. The other foot functions as a balance point.

You can also do this exercise holding on to a couple of dumbbells but because of the angle, you'll need to use very heavy dumbbells to get a decent effect. It's doable but not as good as a barbell.

No excuses for giving up on your calves when you've got a home gym now!

"STAIR-STEPPING" CALF RAISES

This is a very strange-looking calf exercise that is actually incredibly effective for getting a pump in the calves. The reason you actually WANT to get a pump in the calves is that there is a tremendous amount of connective tissue in the lower area (a.k.a. fascia). In order to give the muscles room to grow, you need to actively stretch the fascia.

This is best done by first filling the muscles with blood and THEN doing a hard stretch on the muscle, to give that fascia something to work against with the stretch (like squatting down in a pair of tight jeans right out of the laundry).

So what you're going to do with this exercise is simple: you're going to put a light to moderate weight on the standing calf raise machine, then get into position as normal.

Now, instead of doing a normal calf raise, you're going to do a stair-stepping movement. If you've seen those portable stepper machines, it's the same idea, only you're going to step up and down with resistance on your shoulders.

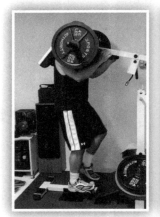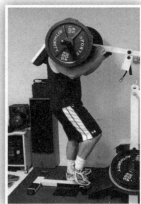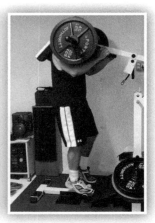

This constant pumping action drives a lot of blood into the calf muscles, even if you normally have a hard time getting a pump in them.

When you've gone as long as you possibly can, give the calves a few seconds rest to allow blood to rush into them. THEN use the calf machine to get a weighted stretch on the calves, holding for as long as you can stand it.

This technique, while it doesn't directly build the calves, sets the stage for future calf growth by helping stretch out the fascia surrounding the calves.

If your calves have been stuck in size, this is a great technique to try. You can even work this into every workout you do, finishing with one set of this.

CHEST

ANCHORED LEGS ONE-ARM DUMBBELL FLOOR PRESS

This is a killer exercise, especially if you're a Mixed Martial Arts fighter, wrestler or other martial artist and you need to train and develop your body to exert power and leverage while you're on your back on the ground.

It's also GREAT training for the lower abs, adductors, and chest all at the same time.

It's basically a One-Arm Dumbbell Floor Press done with your feet/legs wrapped around a pole or beam. So instead of pushing with your leg set out to side, you have to use your core and adductors to oppose the force of the dumbbell press and lock your body into the movement.

Once you see it in action, you'll know exactly what I'm talking about. If you're a MMA fighter, this is one you HAVE to try. It'll develop strength and power and train your ability to USE that strength and power when you're on your back covering up with your legs locked around your opponent.

So to do this one, you'll need a solid pole or object (I'm using the upright of my power rack) and a dumbbell. I'm using an 85 pound dumbbell; pick something you can easily do for one-arm dumbbell bench press the first time you try this one. You can move up quickly from there once you get an idea of how the exercise works.

Now, sit with your butt close to the pole and your feet on either side of it. Lay down and slide your butt as close as you can to the pole. Next, lock your legs onto the pole by crossing your feet.

When doing this one, I like to have my working side leg hooked over top of the other leg, e.g. pressing with the right arm, lock the right leg over the left, around the pole.

Now reach over and grab the dumbbell with both hands to get the weight into position.

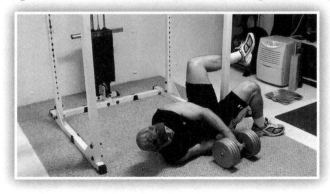

Hold the dumbbell on your chest and get it into your right hand.

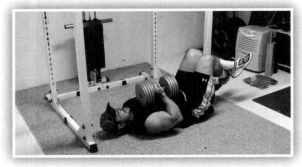

Bring your right arm down and out to the side, with your upper arm on the floor.

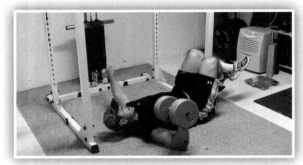

Tighten the clamping of your legs HARD then get ready to press. Your left arm is out to the side for balance.

Press the dumbbell to lockout. This is the hard part and the reason why you should start light It'll take some serious tension in your adductors and lower abs to keep your body straight while pressing the dumbbell up.

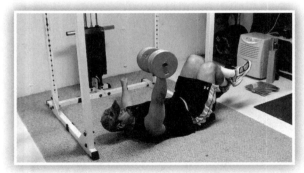

Do four to six reps on one side, lower the dumbbell to your chest, and switch hands. Switch your feet over at the same time so your left leg is locked over the top.

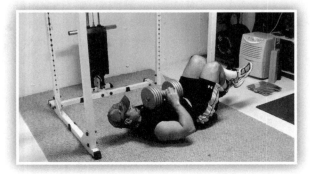

Now get the dumbbell off to the side and go again.

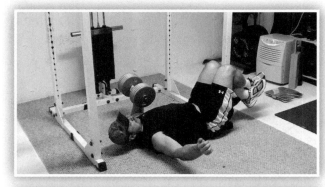

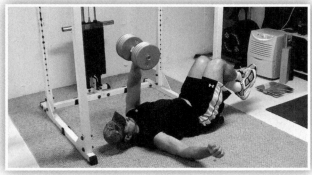

That's the exercise!

As you can see, this is a PERFECT exercise for developing ground-strength for MMA fighting. You'll be developing power when flat on your back with your legs wrapped around something and you'll learn how to USE that power.

If you're not a MMA fighter, this is a great core and adductor exercise in general. It's not going to hit your chest incredibly hard because you're forced to use a lighter weight than you could use for normal pressing, but chest development isn't really the goal of this one anyway; it's the ground-based power development.

BACK-OFF-BENCH DUMBBELL PRESS

The bench press: a key movement for your chest that, ironically enough for some people, doesn't even work their chest all that well!

THIS version of the dumbbell bench press is going to force continuous tension on your chest while placing

TREMENDOUS tension on the abdominals as well (you'll see why in a second).

The Back-Off-Bench Press is a unique movement for the chest that LOOKS like a standard dumbbell bench press, until you look a little closer. You'll be doing the bench press with your upper back hanging off the end of the bench!

And while it is true that you'll be forced to use less weight than in a normal bench press, I found this technique basically FORCED the pectoralis muscles into continuous tension. I got a GREAT pump using lighter dumbbells and hit the core at the same time (especially the rectus abdominus six-pack muscles). This is the ideal beach body exercise: chest, abs and arms all in one shot

Don't let that "beach body" thing fool you though; this exercise is VERY tough and actually very valuable. It's definitely one I'm going to be including in my training more often.

To perform this one, you'll need a few things for the set up: dumbbells (they don't need to be heavy), a bench, and something to brace your legs under. I used a power rack with a loaded barbell set on the rails to brace my legs

on and that worked perfectly (a Smith machine will actually be useful for this). You can also use just about anything else you can think of that you can brace your legs under, even a partner pushing down on your knees, if that's what you've got.

Here's what my setup looked like: a flat bench inside the power rack with the barbell set in the rails at about hip height. You'll need to adjust the bench position under the bar, depending on how it feels when you're doing the exercise. I've got the bar over the midpoint of the bench.

The first time you do this, start with a LIGHT weight until you get a feel for the exercise. If you're using the rack setup, just set a couple of plates on the bar to keep it from coming up.

This is one of the ONLY times I'll ever recommend you set your feet on a bench for bench pressing. In a normal press, you need the stability of your feet on the floor. In this version, your knees will be locked under the bar, giving you stability there.

Grab your dumbbells. I'm using a pair of 65 pound dumbbells in the demo here.

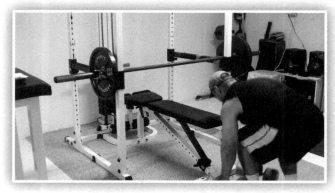

Stand up and set the dumbbells on your hips.

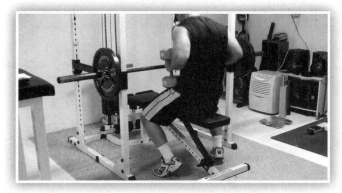

Sit down on the bench and shuffle forward so that your hips are a bit closer under the bar. Again, you'll need to experiment to get the position right for you.

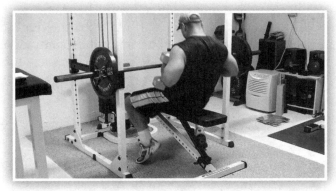

Raise one leg up and brace it under the bar. Then get the other leg up. If you've got a partner to hand the weights to you, this will be even easier; just get into position on the bench first, then have them hand the dumbbells to you.

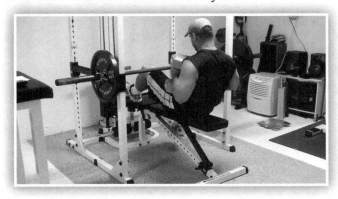

Lay back on the bench and feel where your upper back is. With the moderate weights I'm using, I had the end of the bench right in the center of my shoulder blades. Make sure you have at least that much of your upper back off the end of the bench.

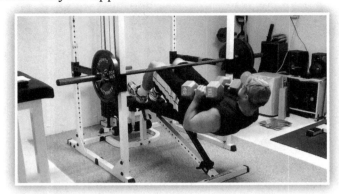

Now bring the dumbbells back and into position for the bench press. THIS is where your abs are going to fire HARD and stay contracted HARD for the duration of the exercise. It's also the reason why the pecs are going to be contracted continuously; your back has nothing to brace against. Therefore, even at lockout the pecs are forced to contract to stabilize and hold the weight.

Taking the back support away places HUGE demands on the entire upper body.

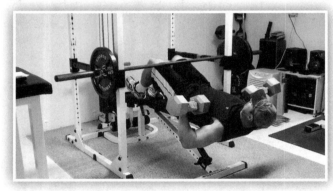

Now press up. Do this exercise at a moderate pace, under control the whole way. You're using lighter weight so go for FEEL with this one and squeeze the pecs at the top. Your abs will contract no matter what you do.

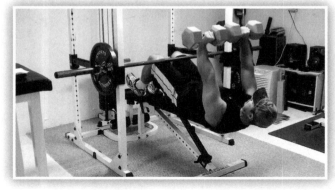

The first time you do this, the weight will be something you'll need to adjust. Go up to about half of what you'd normally use for a heavy set of dumbbell bench press and do six to eight reps.

When you're done, you can either just drop the weights to the floor (which most gyms don't like), or move them back up onto your thighs and use your knee-bracing to do a sit-up.

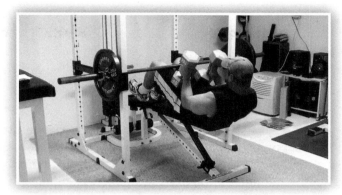

Then just stand up and set your dumbbells down and you're good.

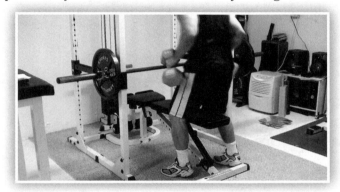

That's the exercise!

Like I said, try it with a lighter weight the first time you do it but definitely give it a try if you've got the equipment. I was very impressed with how powerfully this targets the pecs and the core.

It's a nice alternative when maybe your joints are a bit beat up from doing heavier benching and you still want an intense pec workout.

DIP BELT WEIGHTED PUSH-UPS
IN THE POWER RACK

The push-up (also known as the press-up) is the first exercise you think of when you think of bodyweight training. It's also one of the BEST bodyweight training exercises you can do.

Bodyweight exercises have been shown to increase muscle fiber activation over their free weight and machine counterparts. This means a push-up (assuming equal resistance) would build muscle and strength more effectively than a bench press or machine press.

The main problem with the push-up is that, as great as it is, you are limited by your own bodyweight; there's only so much of you to go around. Granted, there are plenty of variations of the push-up you can use to increase the resistance of the exercise without adding extra weight, but the most straightforward way to increase the resistance is to simply add resistance.

And that gives you several options, several of which require a partner to help you.

1. Have a partner push down or sit on your back.

2. Have a partner load weight plates onto your back.

3. Figure out how to load weight plates or a sandbag onto your back

4. Use a training band over your back and in your hands.

Since I train alone in my basement (my "mad scientist" lab, if you will), I don't have the option of a partner to help me. I've loaded a sandbag on my back, but there is a limit to how heavy of a sandbag you can work with in that fashion. I've also use a training band over the back, which gives nice resistance at the top but zero at the bottom.

To solve all those problems, I now use THIS version: the Weighted Push-Up done with a dip belt, set up in the power rack.

It allows you to very easily set yourself up with as much weight as you can possibly use to load the push-up exercise, which helps with building maximal strength in a way that normal, high-rep push-ups simply can't.

So to do this exercise, you'll need a dip belt and a power rack. Set the safety rails in the power to two different heights: one at hip level, the other at knee level. You'll be setting your feet on the lower one and your hands on the upper one.

The reason we're using two different heights will be apparent when you see the body position of the exercise. Once you've got the rails set, lean some plates up against the rack uprights and get the dip belt on, with the chain strung through the center.

The dip belt should be on your lower back as you get into position.

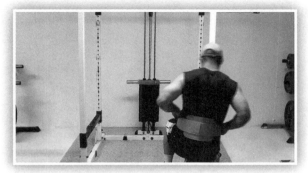

With the plates hanging down, waddle into the middle of the rack (you can't walk normally with weight plates hanging down), lean forward and rest the plates on the ground.

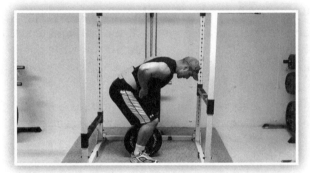

Shift the belt up higher on your back, so it's just below your shoulder blades rather than on your lower back.

This is important in order to move the resistance closer to the arms, which are actually doing the work. If the belt is on your lower back, the movement becomes more awkward and it pulls down on the lower back too much.

The higher belt position gives you more support and allows for greater resistance.

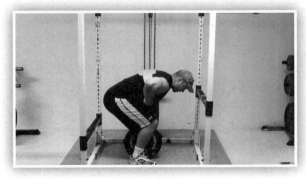

Now get into position, setting your hands on the upper rail at your normal push-up width (for me, it was with my hands against the uprights, since my rack isn't tremendously deep) and setting your feet on the lower rail.

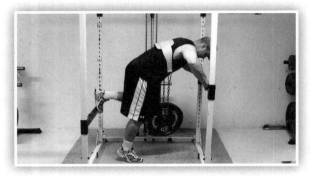

You're ready to begin!

Now here's the reason one rail is lower than the other: we want to keep the torso horizontal during the movement so the belt doesn't slide up or down the back. We also want to keep the body in a pike position, somewhat, as this engages the abs and takes pressure off the lower back.

If you try to keep a straight body position with 180 pounds hanging off you, it will fold you like a burrito. Your body will naturally assume this pike position at the top.

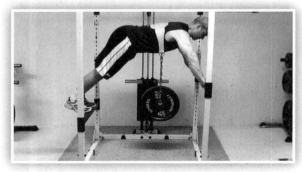

Lower yourself, just like you would in a regular push-up.

As you come down, you will lose some of the pike position, which is totally fine as the weight will actually be pulling forward a bit, taking pressure off the lower back.

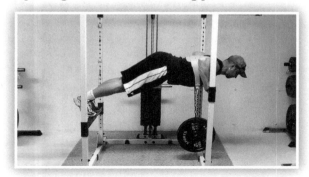

Go down until your chest touches the bar, then push back up, increasing the pike-ness of your body as you come up to protect the back. This does happen naturally, so you probably won't even need to consciously do it.

The first time you try this weighted push-up technique, start with a light weight; don't jump right to your maximum. Get an idea of how to do it, and THEN you can start sensibly increasing the weight from there.

One difference between this exercise and the regular floor push-up is the path of your body. It's not a straight up-and-down movement. This is actually a very good thing, since the angle and arc of the push engages the upper chest more than the lower chest (because you're pushing up and back, away from the safety rail).

If you're strong on the push-up and have been looking for a way to get some serious resistance with it, this is a GREAT way to do it. You can load it to the maximum without needing a training partner to help you.

This is an extremely effective way to develop the pecs with increased muscle fiber activation from a bodyweight and loaded weight exercise .

HOOKED FEET ELEVATED BENCH PUSH-UPS

I f you're looking for a bodyweight exercise that targets the upper pecs, this is a great option for you. It's essentially an incline push-up that takes away one of the biggest problems with that exercise: the floor.

When you do a normal incline push-up (feet up on a bench, body angled down), as you come to the bottom, you have to flatten out your chest in order to keep your face from hitting the floor.

This takes away some of that upper pectoralis focus in the exercise.

So to solve that, you're going to be setting your hands on the front edge of a bench and hook your feet over a bar (or other solid object) to get your body at a downward angle. Because your hands are on the front edge, you're also going to get some additional tension by keeping yourself in place and from gripping the padding of the bench.

To do this one, just set the bench a few feet in front of the bar. I'm using a bar set in the power rack and pulled against the uprights. You can adjust the height of the bar to your liking.

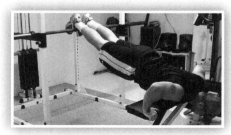

Get your feet hooked over the bar and get your body straight. Now you're in the top position of the push-up.

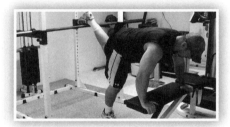

Lower down, push up, then repeat.

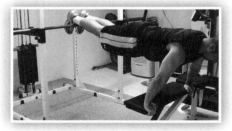

It's a fairly simple push-up variation; the key is what you're setting yourself up on. As you can see in the bottom position, my head is below the level of the bench. This is what allows me to keep that declined body position and maintain tension on the upper pecs.

INCLINE BARBELL BENCH PRESS IN RACK

Training the upper chest is extremely important for overall balance in the upper body, and it's one of the most neglected aspects of chest training, usually for the simple reason that it's harder and you can't use as much weight.

Now, for hitting those upper pecs, the Incline Barbell Bench is one of the most common exercises.

If you're like me, you have a hard time getting results from this exercise when it's done with standard form; all you get are tired triceps and sore shoulders.

If so, I've got the solution for you. It's a very simple adjustment to the setup that you use for the incline barbell press and an adjustment in how you perform the exercise.

One of the biggest problems with the Incline Barbell Bench Press is that the chest and rib cage tend to flatten out during the exercise. This takes the tension off the pecs and puts it on the shoulders and triceps instead.

In order for the pecs to get a good contraction, the shoulder blades need to be pulled tightly in together with the shoulders back and chest and rib cage expanded.

With each rep of the "normal" incline barbell bench press, when you're at the top of the movement (especially when you get the bar off the rack), the full extension of your arms very quickly causes your shoulder blades to come forward and your rib cage to flatten out.

There's no real opportunity to get the shoulders back and behind you again before you start the next rep, so when you lower the bar, the chest is flat and the shoulder blades aren't retracted, taking the emphasis off the pecs and putting it on the shoulders (at the bottom) and triceps (at the top).

And really, just by getting the bar off the rack, you're immediately putting your body in a poor biomechanical position to perform the exercise if the goal is emphasis on the upper chest.

Granted, in a lot of people, they will still get a decent amount of stimulation on the upper pecs, even in this situation; these are the people with more favorable anatomical levers, i.e. they'll feel it in the chest no matter how their arms and shoulder blades line up.

For many (me included), performing the incline barbell press in this position simply doesn't work.

SO HOW DO YOU FIX THE INCLINE BARBELL BENCH PRESS?

It's not hard to do! Instead of performing the incline barbell press in the bench designed for it, we'll set up in the power rack using an adjustable incline bench.

Set the bench to about 30 to 45 degrees—you can experiment with what incline feels best to you—and set it inside the rack.

Now here's the part that's going to take some trial and error: set the side safety rails of the rack to where you think the BOTTOM position of the incline press will be on you.

The first time you do the exercise, set the empty bar on the rack just over top of the bench face, and then slide yourself underneath the bar to gauge the position.

The REAL key with this exercise (for those of us with unfavorable biomechanics) is to start from the BOTTOM and do SINGLE reps, resetting your body position each and every time you are about to press the bar up.

I had pretty much given up on the incline press as completely useless for me for quite a few years!

When I started doing the exercise with this technique, I was VERY surprised at how much better it felt and how it actually WORKED the upper chest.

So back to our setup. With just the empty bar on the rails, grip the bar with a slightly narrower grip than you'd use for flat barbell bench.

The bar should be a few inches above your chest when it is resting on the rails. We want a good range of motion but we also are going to be setting the bar down on the rails after each rep in order to reset the shoulder blades and rib cage, so we still want the bar to finish ABOVE the chest.

If the rail height isn't quite right, adjust as needed then check again with just the bar. Once you've got the right height, load up the bar with a moderate weight—something you know you can do—then get back under the bar again.

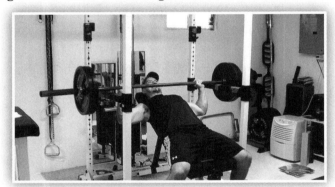

Now here's the next trick: grip the bar and pull your torso just slightly UP off the bench like you're doing a pull-up row. When your torso is off the bench, pinch your shoulder blades together behind your back (just like with a row), puff and expand your rib cage up to meet the bar, then set your torso back down on the bench.

Notice how your shoulders are back, and your chest feels thicker? THIS is the correct position to perform the incline bench press. It's also the position that you usually LOSE almost as soon as you pass the halfway point of the incline press!

Now, with a powerful movement (and striving to keep your shoulders down and back), press the bar off the rails and all the way up in a straight vertical line; there is no backwards arc in the incline bench like there is in the flat bench. It should be straight up and down.

It's important to note that your feet should be dug FIRMLY into the ground, with your knees bent at about

80 degrees. This is because when you press, you want to also push hard with the quads. This locks up the tension in the entire body allowing you to drive that bar up with much more power.

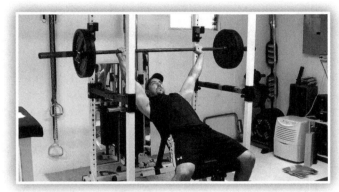

Press it all the way up. You'll notice how as you come to the top, you've probably lost that shoulder position and expanded rib cage. No worries! Lower the bar slowly back down and set it on the safety rails.

Now, RESET your torso, doing exactly what you did on the first rep! Pull your torso up off the bench, get your shoulder blades back, expand your rib cage then set yourself back down on the bench.

Do your second rep the same as you did your first: power it off the rails straight up, then lower it under control back down to the safety rails.

As for rep range, I find this technique lends itself better to lower reps, five to seven reps per set, because of the time it takes to reset yourself between each rep.

At the end of the set, when the bar is back down on the rails, you can either just roll it forward on the rails so you have enough room to slide yourself out from under the bar, or you can duck your head under the bar and sit up again.

This technique is a very effective one for ANY trainer, and especially if you're not particularly biomechanically suited to the exercise. In order to really feel it where you're supposed to, you MUST reset yourself into the best position for your body to perform the exercise: the position that is immediately broken with a conventional un-racking of the bar at the top.

Here's what this setup and execution will do for you:

1. Set your body into the best biomechanical position to perform the exercise on each and every rep, ensuring you're working the actual target muscles.

2. Gives you short breaks in between each rep, which helps you stay stronger during each set, which will allow you to perform more reps with a given weight.

3. Allows you to perform the exercise by yourself, with no spotter, in complete safety.

4. Builds excellent pressing strength out of the bottom because each rep starts from the bottom off a dead stop, with no elastic tension in the muscles.

Give this version a try next time you work chest! You'll notice an immediate difference in strength and tension in the pecs.

LOW PULLEY PUSH-UP CROSS-OVERS...
AND WEIGHTED

This exercise is a deadly combination of three different methods of resistance (and a fourth, which I'll tell you about at the end of the first part).

First, you're going to be doing a regular push-up on your fists—no problem there.

Secondly, you're going to be holding the two low pulleys of a cable crossover machine in your fists while you're doing the push-up. These pulleys will be actively trying to pull your hands apart while you're doing the push-ups, forcing your pecs to contract directly laterally constantly while they're also being used to push your body up.

Third, on each rep, we're going to balance on one fist, and then bring one handle underneath and across your body, similar to a crossover. This is going to add great tension to the extreme inner pectoralis area.

Combine all these into one exercise, and you've got a DEADLY chest movement (that fourth form of resistance is adding on to the push-up via a sandbag on your back, or weight plates, or a partner pushing down).

Here's how to do set it up and do it:

First, set the handles on the low pulleys and set a fairly light weight the first time you do it. Kneel and grab one handle, then go over and grab the other.

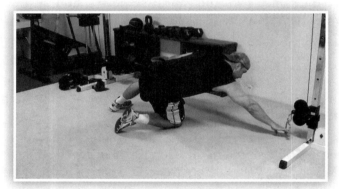

Get into push-up position on your fists; bring the cables into the middle. Set your feet wide to increase your base of support when you're on one fist.

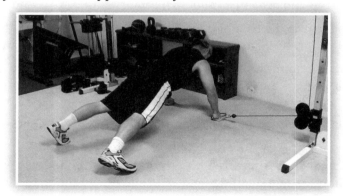

Go down into the bottom position of the push-up, then back up.

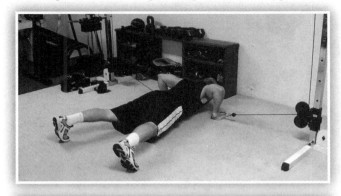

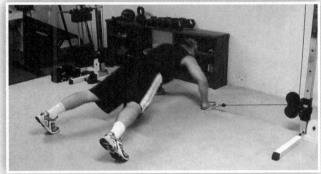

Now the fun part: while balancing on your left fist, bring the right cable underneath and across your body, squeeze and hold for a second or two. This will light up the inner aspect of your pecs.

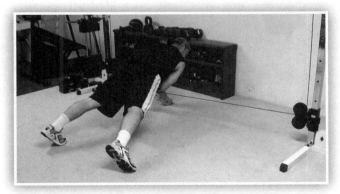

Bring your hand back out and set it down again.

Drop down and do another push-up.

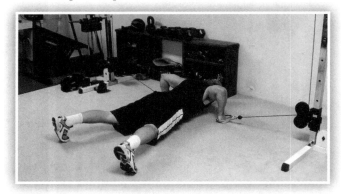

Go back up and bring the OTHER hand under and across and squeeze.

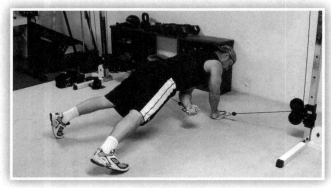

Repeat until your chest is essentially screaming. That's it!

Now, if you're strong enough and want to add even MORE resistance to the movement, this is the next level.

For me, it's a 70 pound sandbag on my back. It's the easiest thing to get into position for doing a weighted push-up. You can use a sandbag or weight plates or a partner pushing down on your back, whatever you have available.

There you have it! This exercise combines multiple resistances to really overload the entire chest.

ONE-ARM BENCH PUSH-UPS

This is a simple variation of the push-up that's going to give you two major benefits:

1. It puts more tension on one arm, similar to a regular one-arm push-up, only it focuses more on the chest than on the triceps, like regular one-arm push-ups do.

2. It puts a great stretch on the other non-working pec muscle as you're coming down into the push-up.

3. You'll be able to use more resistance than just bodyweight, making this exercise more effective for building muscle mass.

Okay, so that's 3 things...

In order to perform this one, you'll need to be able to do at least 15 to 20 normal push-ups, though if you really wanted to, you could potentially do these on your knees, too.

For this, you'll need a bench or a chair or even just stairs; basically anything you can set one hand on that is about a foot and a half off the ground or so. I'm using just a regular flat bench.

Set one hand flat on the bench and the other hand on the floor a short distance away from the bench. Keep your body stiff and straight.

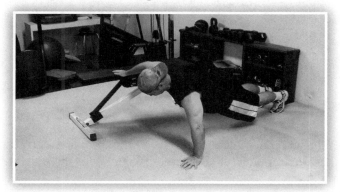

Now lower yourself down, like you would in a regular push-up.

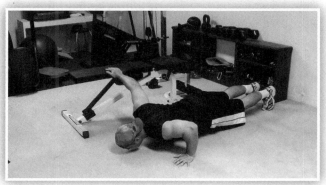

As you can see, my left side is getting the brunt of the load, which works the left pec more. My right arm is placed in a great pec stretching position every single time I come down to the bottom.

The other good thing is that this stretch position is done against resistance (because that pec is also supporting your bodyweight). As you push up, that right pec will also contribute to the movement somewhat, so it's not a true one-arm push-up in which the whole load is on one side.

You get two type of work in one shot, then you switch arms. Same execution.

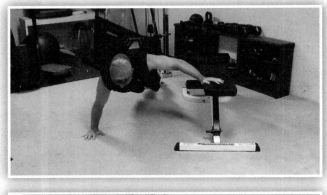

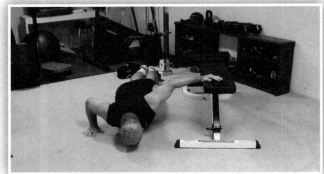

Doing the second side, you'll not get as many reps since you'll already be fatigued from the first. It's fine to take your regular rest period between sides, if you want, in order to keep things more even.

This is a great push-up variation for when you're travelling for a couple of reasons: first, you get more resistance and second, that stretch helps counteract the inwards-pulling position you tend to acquire while travelling (sitting for long periods in a plane or car).

PERPENDICULAR BENCH PRESS

I f you're familiar with the floor press, this is a bench version of that, basically. If you're not familiar with the floor press, it still is, but I'm going to tell you what that means

The floor press is a bench press done while lying on the floor. The reason it's useful is that at the bottom, your upper arms rest on the floor, which allows you to take tension off the pecs so you're starting with zero elastic tension at the bottom of every rep. This helps work the muscles harder because of that missing assistance.

So instead of doing the floor press on the floor, we're going to accomplish the same "zero tension" goal using a bench and that bench will sit perpendicularly to the power rack so that your butt is off in space while your upper back is supported on the bench.

Here's what it looks like:

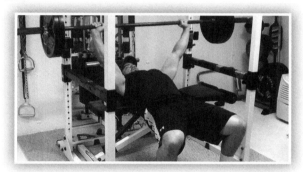

The setup is exactly the same as a regular bench press in the rack except for the bench being perpendicular to the rack and parallel to the bar.

You will find the balance to be a bit different, though, so start lighter than you normally would the first time you do this one. It's actually tougher than it looks and losing the elastic rebound out of the bottom is going to make you work a lot harder.

Un-rack the bar and get it into the top position, as pictured above. Now lower the bar until your upper arms are resting on the bench (instead of the floor). Make sure your safety rails are set so that the bar doesn't come down on them.

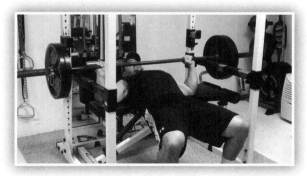

Balance the bar while taking the tension off your pecs, consciously relaxing them. Then regroup, setting your shoulders behind your body (I like to do this by pushing my elbows down into the bench while trying to touch my chest up to the bar—this automatically pulls the shoulders in).

THEN push up with a powerful press out of the bottom.

You'll notice it is a fair bit harder than regular press because you're basically right at the sticking point of the movement at the start point. Developing strength out of the bottom here is going to help you immensely in your full range bench press. You'll blast right through that sticking point.

This is easy to set up and I find it to be easier and safer to perform than floor press, especially if you don't have a good setup to do those and/or no spotter. You get the same benefits but in the protection of the rack.

SHIFTING GRIP BENCH PRESS FOR INNER PECTORAL TRAINING

If you want a better-looking chest (male or female), the inner chest is a key area you're going to want to focus on. It's extremely important from a visual standpoint (think chest cleavage).

The pec is one of the few muscles I've found that you can really effectively develop specific parts of it with targeted angles and movements. This is due to the fan-shape of the pecs; they're designed to move the arms in such a wide variety of directions that you really CAN put more tension on specific areas.

But the inner chest can be tough to really hit effectively with free weight. Not so with this exercise, and I'll tell you right up front: it's a bit evil.

What you're going to do is a set of bench press while shifting your grip first inwards then back outwards DURING the set. The result is EXTREME tension on the inner chest (along with plenty on the triceps as you move your grip in closer).

Here's how it works:

First, set up in the power rack as you normally would for a bench press, with the safety rails just below chest height.

If you're using a free-weight bench station, have a good spotter available to keep an eye on you. You probably won't need one but because of the nature of the exercise, you absolutely SHOULD have one standing by.

Set a light weight on the bar—and by light, I mean LIGHT. I'm using 135 pounds on this one; it's about 50 percent or so of my 1 Rep Max at the time I'm writing this. Trust me, it'll be PLENTY.

In fact, the first time you do this technique, use just the bar, so you get an idea of how to shift your grip easily. Grip the bar as you would for a normal bench press. Un-rack the weight into the top position of the press.

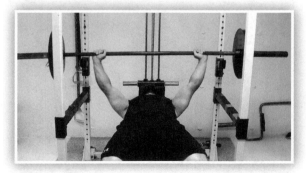

Lower the bar to your chest.

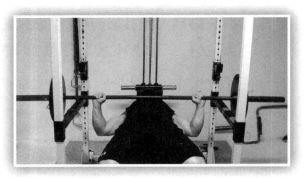

Now the fun begins...

Rest the bar on your chest and shift your grip slightly inwards. I find the best way to do this is to rotate your elbows inward, which shifts where the bar rests on your palms. Then rotate your elbows outward to shift the rest of your hand over. It'll probably move your grip over about a half an inch or so.

The evil part is this: you're doing this shifting while maintaining tension in your upper body and holding your breath, to keep the rib cage and trunk stabilized. It's also one reason you want to use light weight (just the bar the first time). It's not so hard the first few reps but it gets BRUTAL by the end of the set.

The other evil part (yep, there's more than one) is that on EVERY single rep, you're starting from a dead stop. The grip shifting takes away ALL the elastic tension you get in a normal press. This forces the muscles to do all the work, and if you're not used to that, prepare to be humbled.

And I have to say, because of this bar resting, this is actually one bench press version I'm not opposed to a person using a bar pad.

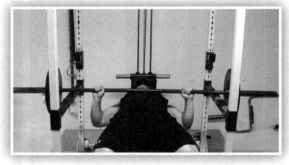

So once you've got your grip shifted inwards a bit, press it up.

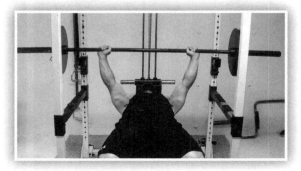

Lower the bar back down then repeat the inward grip shift.

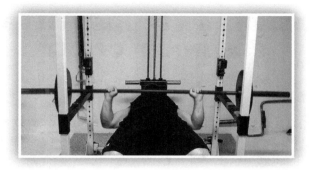

Then press up.

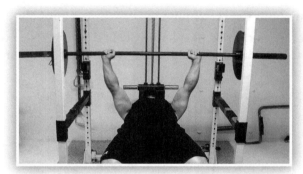

Then lower and shift inwards again. This inwards shifting while under tension helps activate the inner chest aspect, while the closer grip fires them.

Keep repeating this cycle until your hands are in a close-grip bench press position, about shoulder-width apart.

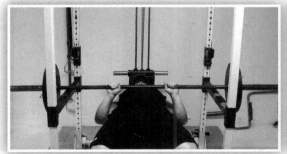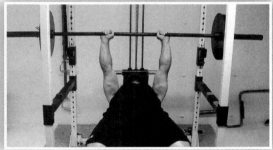

Now for the final evil part:

The close-grip position is the weakest version of the bench press exercise. So to push everything that much further, we're going to shift our hands back OUT to the normal bench press position.

You're going to repeat the same idea as above only doing the opposite, moving your hands outwards.

As you move your hands outward, your pecs will contribute more to the movement and the leverage will get better, allowing you to keep going until you hit that final position.

And you will be VERY happy to hit that final position.

So that's the technique. It's an extremely powerful way to target the cleavage of the inner chest and will light up that area with very targeted tension.

And yeah, it's evil. I admit it.

TILTED DUMBBELL BENCH PRESS
FOR INNER CHEST

I've got a treat for you with this exercise, if you want to fill out your inner chest and get more cleavage of your pecs.

This exercise targets the inner chest fibers very strongly with a heavy press, which is very useful for building, and with very simple equipment (no machines needed, just a decline bench and a dumbbell).

The key to this one is the angle of your body. You'll be lying perpendicularly to the bench with one arm hooked under the roller pads at the top and your shoulders tilting down.

Here's the starting setup: dumbbell beside the decline bench. Use a weight you know you can handle well for normal dumbbell presses. I'm using an 85lb dumbbell here, which is pretty moderate for me.

Sit on the bench and reach down and grab the dumbbell.

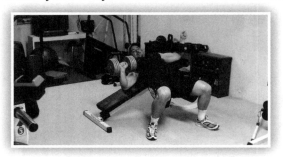

Set the dumbbell on your thigh, and get your other arm hooked underneath the top leg roller pad.

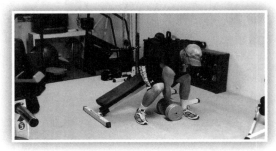

As you do this, kick the dumbbell up into the bench press position.

Now you're in position. Your arm is hooked under and the other arm is in the bottom of the bench press position. Note how my shoulders are tilted down. This is KEY to hitting the inner pec fibers because as you press up, the tilt in your shoulders makes it SEEM like you're coming up and across your body, which is what hits those inner fibers.

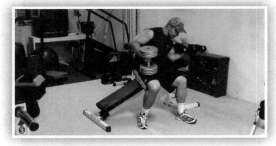

Press up and hold and squeeze HARD at the top. This is not a fast power exercise. You want to do this deliberately and really get that hard squeeze at the top of the movement where your arm comes across your body.

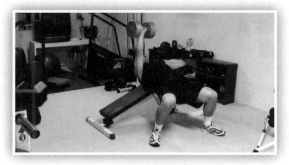

Do all your reps on one side, then set the dumbbell down on the floor and switch to the other side.

You can really see the tilt in the shoulders in this pic. Note how much upper arm is all the way down and practically touching the bench at the bottom; the bottom isn't the "money" part of the exercise, it's the top, so make sure you get that squeeze at the top.

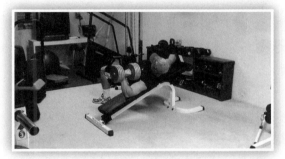

Your bottom shoulder will come off the bench at the bottom, which is totally fine because that's the idea with the exercise. The shoulder comes up as the arm comes up and across.

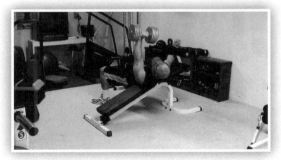

So if you want to hit that inner chest, DEFINITELY give this one a try. It's also going to target your core because of the tilt and the single-arm pressing.

HAMSTRINGS

2 UP 1 DOWN STIFF-LEGGED DEADLIFTS

The Stiff-Legged Deadlift is one of my very favorite hamstring exercises; it can be tricky to learn but the results are worth it.

I've got an advanced version of the SLDL. Only people who are experienced with the SLDL should do this one—it's NOT a beginner exercise.

That being said, you're basically doing negatives with this exercise. The hamstrings are actually DESIGNED for this type of thing (heavy eccentric loading); when you run, every impact your foot makes on the ground your hamstring absorbs the eccentric load .

Not training the hamstrings eccentrically can theoretically lead to them being more prone to hamstring pulls. If you train the hams to absorb and deal with this impact, you'll have a lot fewer injuries.

So for this exercise, you're going to go up with both legs, step one foot back a little, then lower the weight with all the tension on the forward leg. The back toe remains on the ground for balance.

Here's what it looks like:

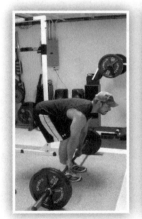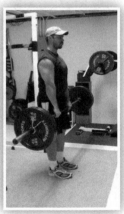

That's the Two-up part. Now for the one down part:

Notice how my right foot is back a bit—there is basically no tension on that back leg. It's all on the front leg.

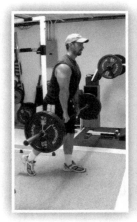 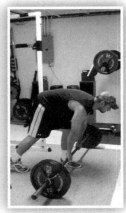

Go all the way to the ground, set your feet together again, and go back up with TWO legs. Then put the other leg back on the way down.

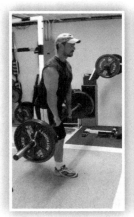 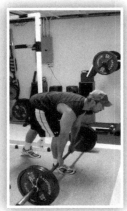

This one is VERY tough. You'll have to experiment a bit with loads to see how much weight you can handle on one leg. I'm using 225 pounds on the bar and I can do normal SLDL's with 400-plus pounds pretty easily.

Remember to keep your lower back arched and your core tight as you're lowering the bar.

If you're an athlete or coach any athletes who do a lot of sprinting or fast running, this exercise is EXCELLENT

for helping to injury-proof the hams.

ANCHORED BARBELL STIFF-LEGGED DEADLIFTS

One of the best hamstring exercises you can do is the Stiff-Legged Deadlift. But it can be a tough one to really feel working properly; you really need to be in tune with the muscle to make the hamstrings do the work.

The reason for this is that when you just use regular free weight, like a barbell or dumbbells, it's tough to keep tension on the hamstrings. There's nothing really for them to work against other than gravity. It doesn't make it a bad exercise, it just doesn't make as straightforward to get the best feeling in the hamstrings.

But when you anchor one end of the barbell, everything changes. You're doing the exact same movement but instead of having everything moving around and having a tough time keeping tension on the hams, you are pulling backwards and leaning against the anchored end of the barbell.

This gives your hamstrings something to work against in addition to gravity!

It's very effective and there are tricks you can use to make it even MORE effective.

First, anchor the barbell end by bracing it in the corner of a machine or wall (once you start getting heavier in weight, you may need to add some weight to that anchored end. Just put a few 10 lb plates on the bar).

Next, straddle the bar and set your feet about a foot and a half apart. Grip the bar with both hands near the weight plates.

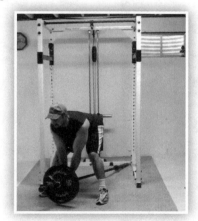

Your knees should be slightly bent but stiff, lower back slightly arched. Once you've got a grip, pull backwards, leaning your weight back against the barbell.

Do a stiff-legged deadlift movement all the way up until you're just short of standing fully upright.

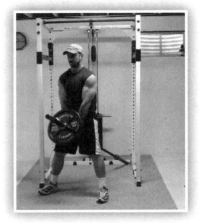

As you lower the bar back down, do it slowly and really lean back against the bar. This puts a great stretch on the hamstrings.

At the bottom, don't let the barbell plates touch the ground in order to keep tension on the hamstrings—that bottom stretch point is the most valuable part of the exercise!

You can also do this exercise with one arm to add in some core work.

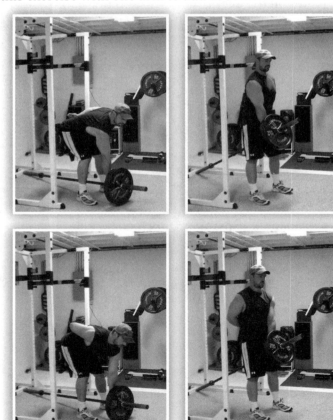

RACK-BRACED DUMBBELL LEG CURLS

If you've ever done concentration curls for your biceps, you know exactly how intense the contraction can be. If you've ever done them without your arm braced against your leg, you know that the contraction can be even stronger. This exercise gives you this kind of intense contraction for the hamstrings. The execution of the exercise also provides a great inner thigh workout!

To do this exercise, you will need a rack.

Start with a fairly light dumbbell to get an idea of how the exercise works and what amount of weight you can use for it.

Set a dumbbell horizontally between your ankles with the front plates at the top of your feet and the handle directly between your ankles and pinch your feet together to support it. It is this pinching that will really hit the inner thighs hard.

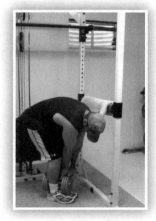

Set the rack safety rail at just above hip height and put a towel over it for padding (or use a bar pad, if you have a round rail).

Push your hips against the rail and set your hands on it. Lean forward and extend your arms to lockout. This will get the dumbbell off the ground.

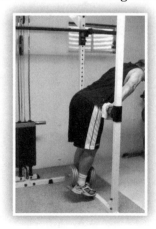

Now do a leg curl with the dumbbell pinched between your feet.

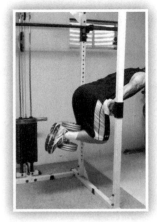

Squeeze hard at the top, then lower slowly and repeat.

Give the Hanging Dumbbell Leg Curl a try on your next leg training day. It's certain to give you one of the strongest contractions you've ever felt in your hamstrings.

HORIZONTAL BAND STIFF-LEGGED DEADLIFTS

I'm a big fan of adding multiple forms of resistance together to better match the strength curve of an exercise, such as using bands to increase the tension on the bench press as you come to the top.

I'm also a big fan of using bands to redirect the tension on an exercise to more closely match the path of an exercise. That might be a bit trickier to understand.

And that's where THIS version comes into play. You're going to be doing a regular barbell stiff-legged deadlift with a band attached to pull horizontally AND vertically (which ends up being diagonally).

I'll explain why it works as I show you the exercise.

First, you'll need a band, a loaded barbell and something to hitch the band on to. I used a bar inside the rack but you don't need to necessarily do that. It could even be the rack itself, but for me, it was out of necessity because that's the best place in my basement gym to do the exercise without banging the bar into anything!

Hitch one end of the band (a medium-tension band is good) to the solid object and put the other end (the loop) of the band over the bar. You don't hitch this end on because you can't hitch two ends of a band and you don't need to. Put the band on before you load the plates on—it's easier that way).

Now stand in front of the bar, grab it and roll it backwards a few feet so you get some stretch in the band to start the exercise.

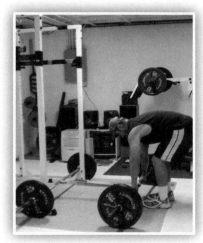

As you can see, you've got stretch right from the start: your glutes and hamstrings are already contracting in order to keep the band from pulling you forward and off balance.

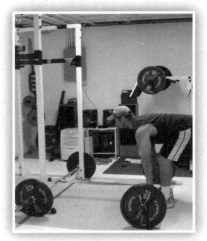

Now begin the SLDL as usual. As you can see in the picture, you still have horizontal tension and not much vertical yet.

Now you're at the top, and you've got more vertical tension and you will lock out against the horizontal (which increases in tension as you come up and back). You can adjust this horizontal tension very easily by either moving yourself a bit closer to or farther from the solid object, which immediately slackens or stretches the band.

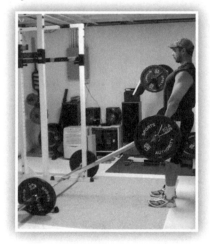

Now just repeat!

Every single rep you do has that gravity resistance and the horizontal/diagonal band resistance to work against. I find this also really works the abs strongly because of how you have to push to keep your balance (core is involved with that) at the same time you're pulling the bar off the ground.

Once you're done, just set the bar down and let the band roll it forward a bit.

THE NEXT LEVEL

Now we come to something a bit more nuts that I tried just to see what would happen, and it really works well! Bit tougher to get set up but it adds even more tension to the hamstrings.

The original band setup is exactly the same: one end hitched, the other looped.

Now you're going to add ANOTHER band. Hitch it to the solid object near the first band. But don't loop it around anything YET. You should also make sure that the second band is laid out underneath the bar. Use a thicker band for this.

Here's the fun part: set your FEET inside the loop of that second band.

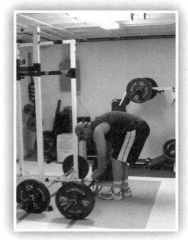

Make sure you get it around both ankles.

Now shuffle backwards. Take a few steps back to stretch the ankle band, and then reach forward and pull the bar back.

Repeat this until you get good tension in BOTH bands. The ankle band is going to be constantly pulling your

feet forward, which you'll have to resist with your hamstrings and core the ENTIRE time you're doing the exercise.

Now perform the exercise as you did before.

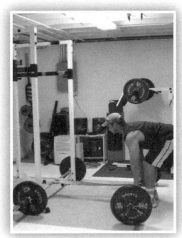

As you can see in the pic below, you get gravity from the free weight, you get diagonal tension from the first band on the movement and you get horizontal tension on your ankles, which adds to the resistance from the other end.

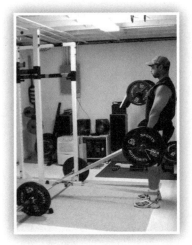

This may look crazy but it really WORKS.

ONE-ARM BARBELL SUMO STIFF-LEGGED DEADLIFTS

This one is a bit of a mouthful, but the exercise name pretty well sums it up. You'll be doing a barbell stiff-legged deadlift in a wide-stance sumo position, using just one arm gripping on the barbell.

This is a GREAT exercise for targeting the lumbar area of the back, not just the middle spinal erector muscles that work in the sagittal plane (straight up and down—imagine a saw cutting your body into left and right halves; movement in that direction is in the sagittal plane), but also the lower back muscles that work to prevent rotation of the spine and torso (anti-rotation).

Working these muscles is much better done by using them to work AGAINST rotation, not to actually rotate, which is a mistake a lot of people make. Twisting movements aren't great for the spine; resisting twisting is a much better way to go.

And that's what this exercise is all about. You'll be lifting the barbell in a standing stiff-legged deadlift movement using just one arm, which puts uneven torque on the core/lower back. This forces those anti-rotation muscles to work hard to keep the body from twisting.

This is a great way to train and strengthen those muscles.

So first, load up your barbell. Start fairly light to get an idea of the movement and how it feels before moving up in weight.

Set your feet out wide in a sumo stance with your toes angled out. The nice thing about the sumo stance is that it keeps your knees out of the way of the bar and makes the exercise a bit easier on the lower back. I find this wide stance really forces the hamstrings and glutes to activate strongly as well.

Grip in the center of the bar with one hand. I recommend using grip assistance with this one as you go heavier. It can be tough to hold on to the bar as you start moving up in weight.

My favorite accessory for this is 1 Ton Hooks.

Keep your knees slightly bent and make sure you have an arch in your lower back. Tighten your core and lift the bar off the ground.

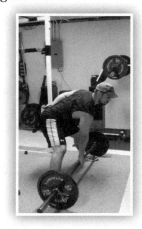

At this point, you'll find out pretty quickly if your grip is positioned correctly, depending on if the bar stays level or tips. If it tips, lower it back down and adjust your grip, then go again.

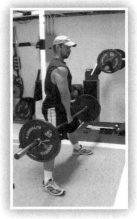

You won't be able to come up all the way to the full lockout that you're used to with the two-arm version. No worries, though, as you'll be getting plenty of work on the lower back even so.

Repeat for your reps on one side (four to six—keep it in the low range for these), and then switch to the other hand.

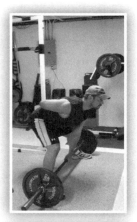

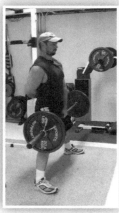

On the next set, start with whichever hand you worked second on the first set, so you keep it even in terms of fatigue and workload.

This is powerful exercise for targeting not only the anti-rotational muscles of the lower back but also the deep core muscles as well, such as the transverse abdominus and the oblique muscles.

The uneven torque on the core forces substantial muscle activation to stabilize the spine, which is why it's so important to start light and work your way up on this one.

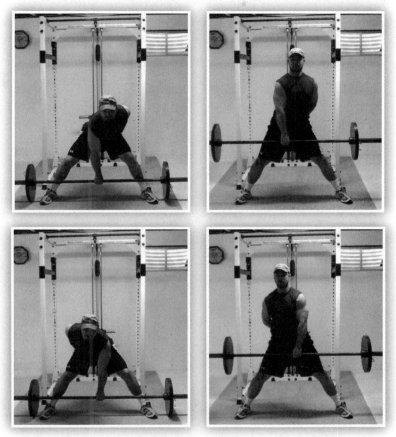

ONE LEG GLUTE/HAM EXTENSIONS

This exercise is a nice one for hitting the two major functions of the hamstrings in addition to the glutes in one movement. I used the power rack rails to do this one but you can use a couple of benches or a bench and some other solid object. It'll be easy to adapt to whatever equipment you have available once you see what it looks like.

I'll use the rack as the explanation since that's what I'm using in the demo here.

Set the rails a few feet off the ground. I have a towel set over the one that I'll be resting my upper body on. The other rail should be set at the same height. Put your back on the rails.

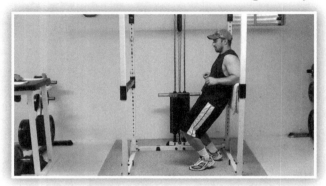

Now rest your elbows on the rail with your mid-back resting against the rail. Set one foot on the other rail. The forefoot area of your shoe should on the top corner section of the rail as your foot will be rolling up and onto the rail as you do the exercise.

Take your other foot off the floor, and let your working leg straighten out.

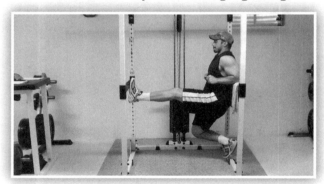

Now use hamstring power to lift your body up. Your knee will bend at this point and this lower part of the movement targets the knee-flexion function of the hamstrings.

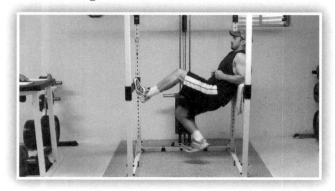

As you come up, the pivot of the exercise will change and your hips will straighten out. Push your hips up as high as you can and squeeze the glutes. This hip extension also is a function of the hamstrings, in addition to targeting the glutes.

Your back will roll up and over the railing here.

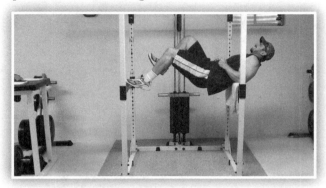

Do three to five reps on one leg, then switch to the other.

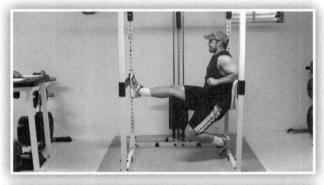

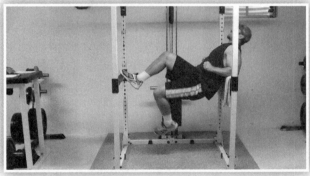

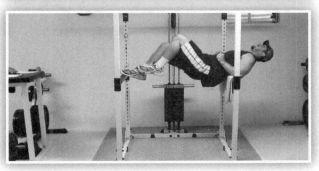

If you need extra resistance, you can hold a dumbbell in your hand while doing the exercise.

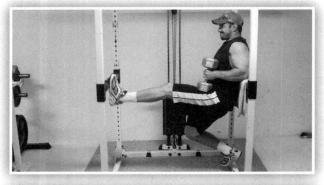

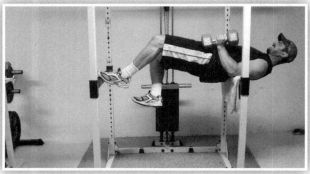

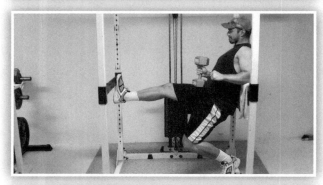

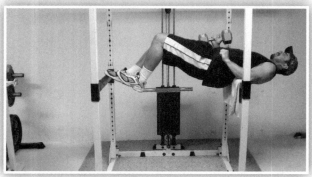

As you can see, it's not an easy one to do but it's a GREAT hamstring exercise that you can do with very little equipment and that doesn't put stress on the lower back like a stiff-leg deadlift can.

It's a nice one if you don't have access to much equipment for training your hamstrings.

STAGGERED STIFF-LEGGED DEADLIFTS

For developing hamstrings, there's not much better than a good Stiff-Legged Deadlift. THIS is a great variation of it.

Basically, you're going to get the advantages of a regular stiff-legged deadlift (the ability to use a good amount of weight) AND the advantages of a one-legged stiff-legged deadlift (focus on one leg at a time).

I like this exercise for athletes; especially those who have to lunge forward and then pull back, e.g. tennis.. But honestly, any athlete who places high force requirements on the hamstrings is going to benefit from this one. The uneven pull on the body is really beneficial.

So load the bar with about half of what you'd normally do for barbell SLDL's (to start with).

You can start one of two ways with this exercise. You can go directly to the staggered position right out of the bottom; all you do is set one foot a bit back from the other. In the demo, I have my right foot toes in line with the heel of my left foot.

You don't want much separation here.

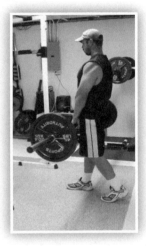

Here's the bottom position.

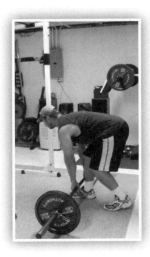

Basically, it's the same exercise as the regular SLDL only you have your legs a little staggered. The balance is a bit different, too. Your front leg is going to have the primary tension on it.

I like to do one or two reps, then switch to the other leg forward.

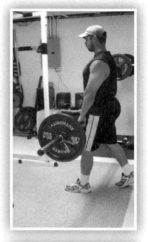

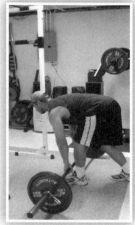

This is a great alternative to normal Stiff-Legged Deadlifts. It provides a nice challenge to the hams and, when you talk about "functional" exercises, it doesn't get much more functional than this.

WEIGHT PLATE LEG CURLS

This is a great hamstring exercise when you don't have access to a leg curl machine. It combines not only the knee flexion function of the hamstrings (bringing your heel to your butt), but how you perform this particular exercise also incorporates the hip extension function of the hamstrings, which is something the leg curl exercise misses.

For this, you just need a weight plate. I'm using a 45-pound plate in the demo. Set it on the floor about five feet away from something solid you can grip. I'm in the rack for this one but it doesn't matter what you use.

Now lie down and grab on to that solid object with your feet on top of the weight plate. I hook my heels in the edge of the plate.

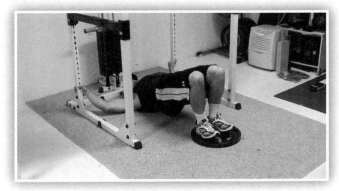

Push the weight plate forward, sliding it along the floor. It's best to do this exercise on carpet, if you can. Rubber flooring will be tougher to slide on.

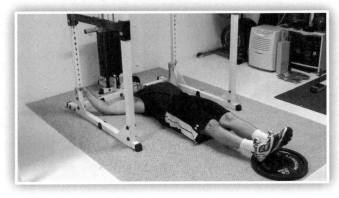

Now PULL the weight plate back and up towards your butt while at the same time pushing your hips UP towards the ceiling.

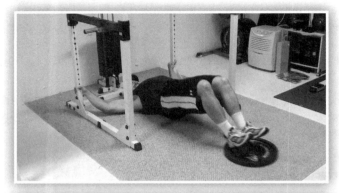

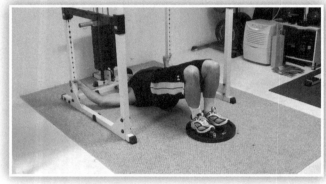

I like to use an explosive movement for this one because that's really what the hamstrings are designed for.

And believe me, the contraction you get from this one is HUGE. You're combining the two functions of the hams into one movement, which really makes for an intense exercise.

This is a great one for home trainers who don't have access to a lot of machines and who need something beyond stiff-legged deadlifts for their hamstrings.

QUADRICEPS

4X RESISTANCE SQUATS

This exercise is the result of an experiment in insanity (unlike everything else I've written about in this book, of course.)

One day I decided to see how many different forms of resistance I could use on a single exercise: the squat. You can apply the principles at work here to exercises with whatever equipment you have available to you; even two forms of resistance is powerful stuff!

Normally, you would think that one form of resistance would be good enough and all you'd need to do is load more weight on to make it harder. That IS true to a certain point, but most exercises (even the squat) don't fully overload the body through the whole exercise.

I've found that by combining different forms of resistance, you can properly overload the entire strength curve of an exercise. In the case of the squat, it's tougher at the bottom and gets easier as you come to the top. Nothing surprising there—anybody who's done a squat knows that.

So, I set up the squat machine with a moderate amount of weight, and set two moderate-weight dumbbells underneath. That's two.

Then I took two training bands and attached those around the weight posts and the footplate of the machine. That's three.

Finally, I put on my 85-pound weight vest and wore it during the squat. That's four.

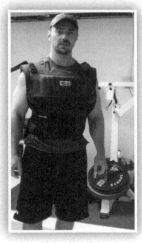

The result? AMAZING overload to the entire body on this exercise.

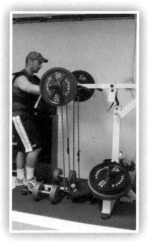

Here's the bottom of the squat. At this point, it's just dumbbells and weight vest providing resistance. The squat machine only kicks in halfway up and because the bands are attached to the squat machine, they don't kick in until the machine is used.

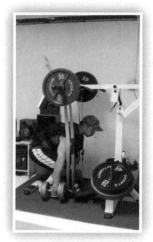

The halfway point—I'm now lifting against the machine as well. The bands are just starting to stretch.

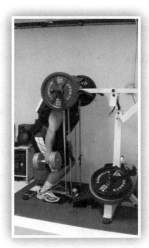

Full lockout. At the point, you've got all four types of resistance pushing down on you. And as the bands stretch, the harder it gets as you come to the top, which is exactly what you want for the squat.

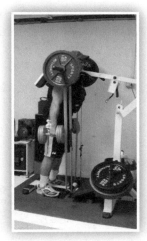

The best part? Not only do your legs get worked, but because you're also holding two dumbbells and wearing a weight vest, your upper body and core gets a tremendous workout as well (much more so than with conventional squats).

Now I know you most likely don't have ALL the equipment to do all four types of resistance but if you've got two or even three, give this exercise a shot. And if you've got all four, say hi to the floor for me because that's where you'll be at the end of the set!

BAR-IN-FRONT WALKING LUNGES

I'll be straight with you: REAL quality leg training is TOUGH. It hurts and it's uncomfortable.

And if you want great legs, you MUST put in the time using challenging exercises such as squats, lunges and variations of the two (leg press is ok and optional).

So on that note, I've got a deadly variation of the Walking Lunge exercise that will push your legs to the EDGE. I call it the Bar-In-Front Walking Lunge.

And the reason I call it that is because that's what it is; you'll be doing a standard Walking Lunge exercise holding the barbell in front of you rather than putting it on your back or holding dumbbells.

This use of the barbell has several advantages:

First, you don't need a rack or a spotter to get the bar in position on your back for a barbell lunge.

Secondly, if you train at home and your dumbbells aren't heavy enough (or if you don't have any) and if you don't have a squat rack or spotter, then this is a GREAT exercise for targeting the legs. When you train at home with limited equipment, it can tough to find exercises that really challenge the legs that you can do without safety equipment like a rack. This exercise is it.

Third, holding the long Olympic bar is good for balance when doing the exercise. If you've ever seen a tightrope walker holding a giant pole while walking, it's a similar concept.

So first, load a barbell with a weight you can pick up and carry fairly easily. I've got 135 pounds on the bar. Grip with a moderately wide grip; I have my pinkies on the smooth ring of the bar. A narrower grip will give you less control over the bar while too wide will make your grip give out before your legs are fully worked.

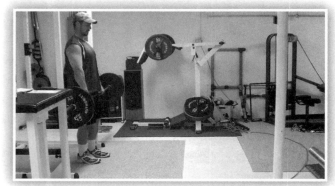

Stand up with it.

Now take a step forward, coming down into the lunge position. At this point, the bar will be resting on your thigh, as close in to your body as you can set it.

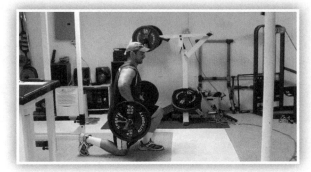

Now stand up pushing up and forward, bring the bar up with you.

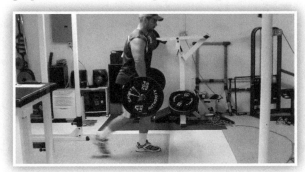

When doing a Walking Lunge, you can either pause at the point and stand on two feet and get your balance before stepping forward again or you can just take another step forward without setting your other foot down. That's the way I like to do it—definitely more challenging.

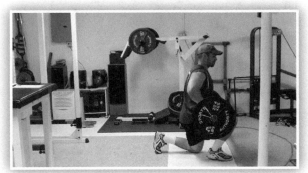

Come down into the next step, again, resting the bar on the thigh at the bottom.

When you've gone as far as you can in one direction, set the bar down, step over to the other side of it, and pick it up and go back.

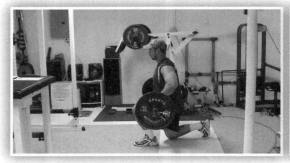 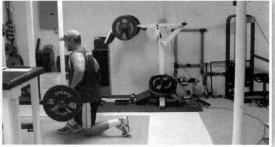

In this view, it's easier to see where the bar is set: right up close to the body. The arms are bent as you come down.

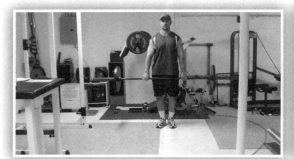 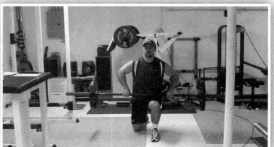

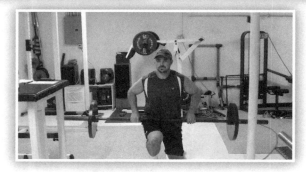

Keep going until you're back to the original start position.

Then turn around and go again, if you have it in you! This will depend on how much weight you're using, your leg endurance and your grip strength.

I can promise your legs will be a quivering mess by the time you're done and you will be breathing extremely heavily. Walking Lunges are extremely good for the legs and for the lungs.

You can use this as a finishing exercise for your leg workout (you won't be keen to do much more for legs after a few rounds of it) or as a mainstay of your leg training, especially if you train with limited safety equipment.

I like to go for distance-reps on this one, going four times back and forth, for example.

BARBELL CURSING LUNGES

Yes, this may be a unique name for an exercise, but the first time you do this exercise, you'll know EXACTLY why I called it that (the other name I had in mind was "Evil Bastard Lunges").

Basically, you're going to be doing what looks like a hack lunge with a barbell (like a lunge holding the barbell behind your back instead of on your shoulders). That's about the best way to describe it. But it's got some key points that take the exercise from a mere lunge to something that will light a fire in the quads that will leave you on the floor—pretty much every set I did ended with me falling down.

You can also do this exercise in a rack, which will allow you to really push your legs HARD and maximize the effect of the exercise. It's not necessary, though, and you can do it very effectively freestanding with just a barbell.

Stand with the barbell behind you, squat down and grab it with an overhand grip (I grab it about the same width as for bench press, using the smooth rings as a guide).

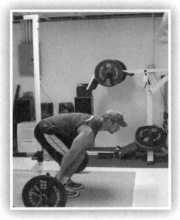

Once you've gripped the bar, stand up, bringing the weight up behind you so that it's resting on the backs of your thighs.

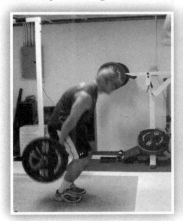 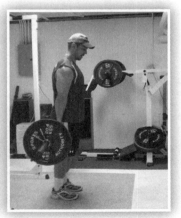

Now step your left leg forward into a typical lunge stance.

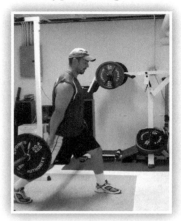

Go down into the lunge with the barbell resting on the back of your right thigh (your back leg,).

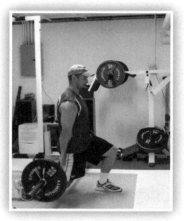

Now the fun begins: instead of standing upright, keep your torso leaning forward. And as you stand up and straighten your front leg, straighten your back leg, PUSHING THE BARBELL UP AND BACK as you do so.

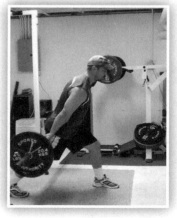

Basically, even though your left leg is forward, it's the RIGHT leg that is actually working directly against the resistance of the barbell. The harder you push to straighten your leg, the stronger the contraction you'll get in the quads.

You're supporting the entire weight of the barbell on your thigh, and quad contraction is what's keeping it there. The left leg gets some work but nearly as much as the right leg; the back leg is the one to really focus on.

And here's the beauty of it: at the bottom of the lunge, when your right leg is bent, you're actually putting a good STRETCH on the right quads as well.

THAT is the reason I call this the Barbell Cursing Lunge. The quadriceps of your back leg gets NO break through the whole exercise from stretch to contraction and through the ENTIRE set.

With a regular lunge or squat, when you come to the top, your skeleton is supporting the weight, not your muscles. It's tough to keep a contraction without shortening the range of motion.

With this exercise, the more you try to lock out at the top, the stronger contraction you'll get in the quads and the harder the exercise will work you.

Take my word for it, it's a serious experience in leg training and it'll really open your eyes. It blew my mind when I came up with it.

And THAT is the reason I'm telling you to do this exercise in the rack: because when you're done, you're DONE. Your leg will give out from the burn and you'll have to set the weight down. The shorter the distance the barbell has to go, the better.

Having the bar a little higher up at the start also makes it easier to begin the exercise, which helps a lot. Here's how the other leg looks (quick tip: because BOTH legs get worked even though the back leg is doing most of it, the second leg you do is going to be quite a bit harder! If you like, you can rest for a minute, then do the other leg instead of doing both at once).

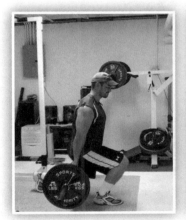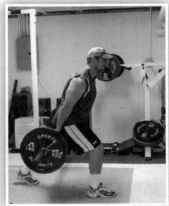

BACK VIEW

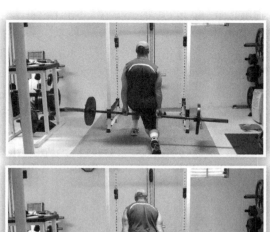

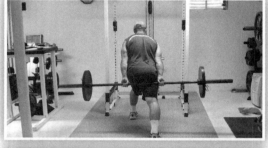

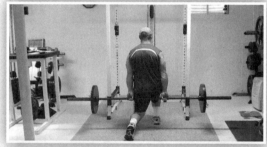

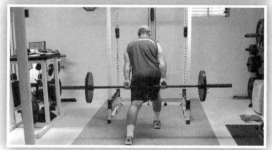

Here's the view of the exercise done using the safety rails of the rack.

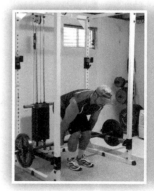
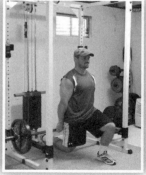
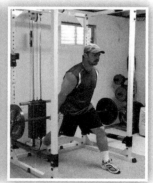

BRACED LEG SQUATS

W hen it comes to working the quads, there's nothing better than the squat. But if your goal is ONLY working the quads and not much else in the lower body, you might turn to leg extensions.

But here's the problem: leg extensions can be trouble for your knees, especially if you already have bad knees, or if you use a ballistic movement on the exercise, or too much range of motion. Clearly, the leg extension can really work the quads hard, but sometimes the potential knee issues aren't a good tradeoff.

So what do we do to work ONLY the quads then? The Braced Leg Squat.

This exercise locks the lower legs into place during the squat movement. What this does is send the VAST majority of the tension of the exercise directly into the quads. It's almost like doing an inverse leg extension, but instead of the thighs being locked down and the lower legs moving, the lower legs are locked down and the thighs are moving.

This exercise uses the same concept of locking down the lower legs, but is done using only a bar and a power rack (and a barbell pad, if you've got one), which makes it a lot more accessible.

It's a great exercise and REALLY tough on the quads; if you like a good quad burn, this one will leave you on the floor.

HOW TO DO IT:

The first thing you need to do is set up the bar in the rack. Set the safety rails of the rack near the bottom, probably about 18 inches off the floor. You'll have to experiment with heights to get the right spot for you.

I like to use a barbell pad on the bar for cushioning. A towel wrapped around the bar will work, if you don't have a pad available. Set that right in the center of the bar. Set the bar on the rails and brace it against the uprights of the rack. I'll explain the exercise without weight first but you can do it holding onto dumbbells as well.

It's CRITICAL that you have on shoes that grip well to the floor for this exercise. Your feet aren't going to be braced against anything; only friction and muscle power are going to be holding them in position.

Step into the rack and set your feet right in front of the bar. Your upper calves (just below the knees) should be braced against the barbell. Your heels should be right underneath the bar, and, your shins should NOT be vertical but at a bit of a forward-leaning angle. This slight angle will help to lock your lower legs into the movement because instead of your feet being able to slide forward, the slight angle means they have to dig into the floor before they can slide forward—even that slight angle helps a lot.

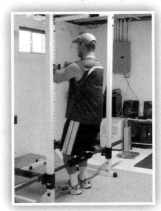

Hold your arms either straight out in front of you or crossed across your chest, whichever you prefer.

Now sit down! Keep your torso vertical and drop back like you are doing a squat. Because your lower legs are locked into position, your knees will be the pivot point. It may sound like it could hurt the knees but in my experience there is a LOT LESS stress on the knees with this one than with leg extensions.

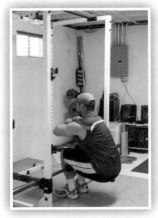

Go down until the tops of your thighs are parallel with the ground. Then, squeezing your quads hard, go back up all the way to the top. I like to come to full vertical and relax the quads for a moment to let some of the lactic acid dissipate. You can keep tension on by not coming all the way up but, believe me, there will be no shortage of lactic acid or tension even if you DO come all the way up.

At this point, you may find you need to readjust your foot position to get the best feel for the exercise; it's hard to get it exactly right on the first rep. So fix your foot position if you need to, and then sit back down and repeat!

To add resistance to this exercise, hold a pair of dumbbells.

You can hold them beside your body with your arms hanging down or in the top of the curl position. Each position puts slightly different tension on the quads. Try both to see which you prefer.

HANGING POSITION:

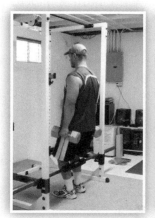 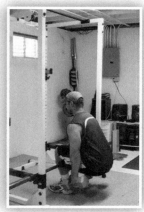

GOBLET POSITION:

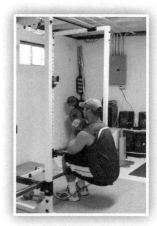

I've also found using dumbbells makes for a great drop set—you literally drop the weight when you can't do any more reps with the dumbbells! At the bottom of the squat, just set the dumbbells down on the floor and keep going using only bodyweight.

When you start getting near the last few reps that you can possibly do, you can also spot yourself by pushing against your thighs. It gives you a bit of help and allows you to keep going.

You'll find with this exercise that the lactic acid really starts cranking up. To flush it out, shake your quads a little at the top standing position to let some circulation help remove some of it. Then keep going!

And if you want another challenge, try dropping the safety rails down one more notch so that the bar hits a little lower on the calves. This allows you to sit even LOWER into the squat because the bar or pad don't get in the way of your hamstrings as you sit down. Squat as far down as you can possibly go with this one—it's a great finisher.

CLOSE STANCE DUMBBELL SPLIT SQUATS

T he dumbbell split squat is one of my very favorite thigh exercises. It really allows you to hit the thighs hard and, when you're toasted, just set the dumbbells down instead of having to re-rack a barbell from your back.

THIS version is the same basic movement but with more of a focus on the quads. You're going to take a very close stance, with your back foot only about twelve inches behind you. Then you'll do the split squat in that position.

This closer stance really puts the focus on the quads. You'll feel a big difference over the standard version. So, grab your dumbbells and hold them at your sides. Then step your right foot back a little.

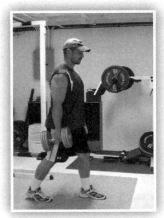

Now squat down. You'll notice that you have to lean forward a bit more than with the regular split squat position. This is totally fine. All part of the fun.

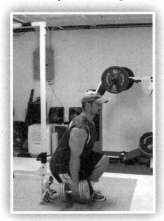

Do all your reps on the right leg, then switch up and put the left leg back. This picture really shows you just how close the feet should be. You can experiment with how far or how close to put them.

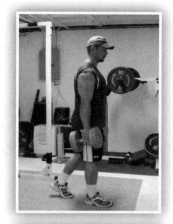

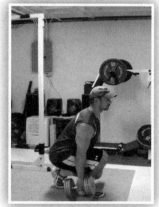

This is a great exercise if your goal is to put the focus on the quads.

DUMBBELL SWITCH LEG SPLIT SQUATS

This is a great leg exercise that really forces the muscles to do the work by taking away any hint of elastic or rebound help out of the bottom of the split squat position. You do this by switching legs in the kneeling position at the bottom of the movement, coming back up on the opposite leg from the one you came down on.

You'll start in a standing position.

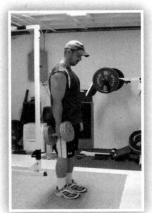

Go down into the bottom position with one leg back—this part is like a Step Back Lunge.

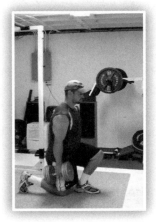

Bring your front leg back and kneel on both knees.

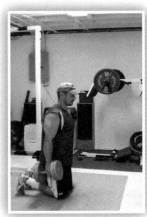

Now bring the other leg forward and get into the split squat position again.

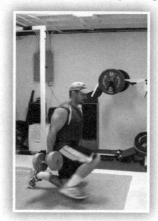

Come up to the standing position again.

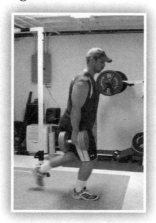

You can do all your reps in one direction before switching, or immediately step back with the same leg and go around the other way.

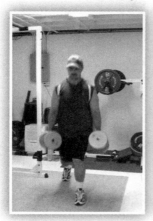 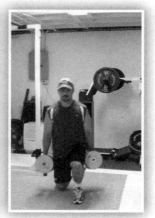

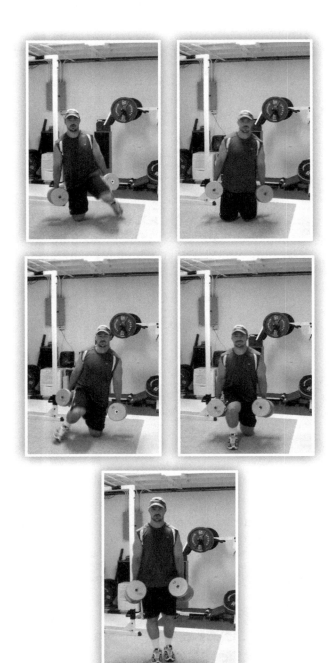

You can also do another variation of this exercise in which at the top, you come up on only one leg and don't touch the other one down. This keeps good tension on the muscles at the top.

Then, just step back and repeat in the other direction, holding your other leg off the ground at the top of the movement.

This exercise in general is a very good one for the legs. It looks like it might be hard on the knees but I haven't found that when I've done it.

LENGTHWISE BARBELL SQUATS

This leg exercise is a whole new animal. I find it to be VERY good for really giving the thighs a beating. Because of how you do it and the set up of the exercise, it's ALMOST like combining the two best features of a squat and a leg press into one exercise.

Once you see how the exercise is done, I'll tell you more about the why and how of that.

First, you will definitely need a power rack for this one. The setup depends on it. Basically, you're going to be in a bent-over position with the barbell running lengthwise down your back. It's tough to explain; pictures will do a better job of it.

This picture shows me getting into position underneath the barbell. For illustration purposes, look at how the rack, barbell and rails are set up. The left hand rail is about three feet or so

off the ground, and the right hand rail is about two feet or so off the ground. This puts the barbell at a downward angle.

I have a foam barbell pad on the bar where my back is going to go (you can use a rolled-up towel for padding here, too). I have the barbell loaded equally: three plates on each side.

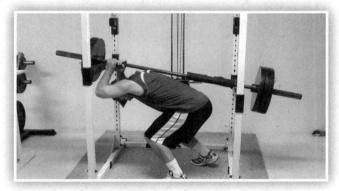

Grip the barbell with both hands where the higher end is resting on the rail. That is going to be the pivot point of the exercise.

Squat down to get your back underneath the lower end of the bar. You'll need to experiment with different rail heights to get the best setup for you.

So then, get yourself underneath the bar with the bar centered down your back. Here's what a direct view of the position looks like. Note that my hands are up by the pivot point and the padded end of the bar is across my lower back.

This may sound like a painful experience, but actually isn't. The barbell is pretty comfortable going lengthwise down the back, even with fairly heavy weight.

So now you're underneath the barbell. Your feet should be pretty wide apart to help you keep your balance.

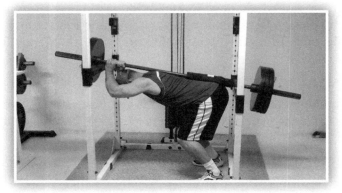

Now straighten your legs, pushing the lower end of the barbell up. The other end should pivot on the other rail, up by where your hands are.

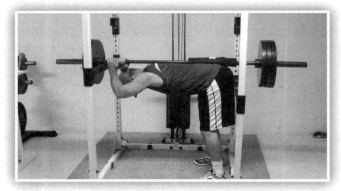

Lower it almost to the rail again and repeat! That's the exercise. Here's a different view of it.

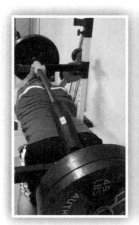 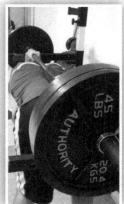

The beauty of this exercise is that you can keep going until your legs are TRASHED, because when they're done, all you have to do is set the bar back on the rails. No getting the weight back into racks, no getting stuck under a huge leg press sled when you push to absolute failure.

This exercise is effective like a squat because it involves moving the body through space rather than like the leg press where you're moving just the weight. Exercises that involve moving the body tend to recruit more overall muscle mass and carry over better to real-world strength. This exercise does that quite well.

It also takes a good deal of stabilizing from the body to do the exercise. The higher end of the bar is basically fixed, but the back end can move very freely. You have to use the thighs not only to move the weight but to control the movement of the bar as well.

At the same time, it's similar to a leg press in that it IS a somewhat fixed movement. You can still concentrate on just pushing the weight (which is an advantage of the leg press) while not having to worry a whole lot about proper technique or if you're going to be able to get the weight all the way back up to the top.

As I mentioned above, this frees you to really focus on destroying the thighs!

The bent-over position of the exercise is more similar to a leg press than a squat, providing you with a very different feel for a bodyweight exercise. If you think about it, a regular leg press is basically the bent-over position, too (90 degrees at the waist). The difference is, of course, you're sitting and not standing.

Put all these things together and you've got one killer exercise!

ONE ARM GRIPPING DUMBBELL SQUATS

This is a great way to get a HUGE range of motion on a squat exercise while keeping your torso in a very upright and neutral position.

Most squat exercises have you freestanding, which means you have to compensate for the position of the weight by basically being less vertical, which puts tension onto the back.

That's not necessarily a bad thing, but it can be an obstacle for some people, especially if you want to get FULL range of motion.

This version is a one-dumbbell squat using the OTHER hand to grip a bar. You can use this grip to spot yourself, but primarily to brace your body. This will allow you to keep your torso more upright while doing DEEP squats.

It's a nice exercise that will let you hit your quads and glutes HARD.

I'm using a 125 pound dumbbell and I've got the bar set on the rails of a power rack about four feet off the ground. You can see how even at the bottom of the movement, my torso is vertical and I'm sitting back. THAT is what this exercise does for you.

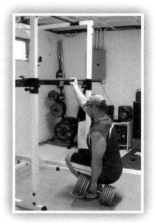

Now just stand up.

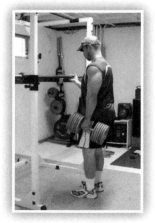

Torso stays vertical the whole time.

I like to do half the reps on one side then immediately switch to the other for balanced effects on the core and legs.

On each rep, don't take tension off the legs, but touch one end of the dumbbell on the ground to make sure you're getting full range of motion. Just keep that tension on!

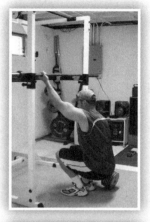

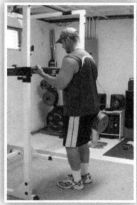

Being able to sit back like this is also going to help you keep your knees from going beyond your toes (if you're worried about stuff like that—me, I'm not worried because the knee is designed for movements like that).

And unless you have knee issues, deeps squats are NOT bad for your knees, as many people worry about. Smith machine squats and leg extensions are MUCH worse for your knees.

This is a nice variation to try; it also allows you to really push the reps until your legs are trashed, since you can just set the dumbbell down when you're done and you can use your arm to spot yourself.

ONE-ARM GRIPPING DUMBBELL SQUATS TO STEP-BACK LUNGE IN-SET SUPERSET

S o this is a pretty complicated name for what is actually a pretty simple exercise, once you understand it.

The In-Set Superset concept is alternating reps of two different exercises that share a similar start or end position. This is done instead of a normal superset doing a full set of one exercise then right into a full set of a second exercise.

I find alternating reps to be an incredibly powerful way to do supersets, much better than regular supersets because of the change in demands on a muscle within the very same set.

So with this one, you'll be doing a single dumbbell squat while holding onto a bar or railing with your other hand. The holding means you can balance and support your body while doing the squat, which allows you to maintain excellent positioning to maximize the effect on the quads. The other hand gripping also allows you to spot yourself, when necessary, to push your legs even harder.

It's a GREAT exercise just on it's own. Now we add a Step-Back Lunge in between reps of that (a.k.a Reverse Lunge).

This is going to target the hamstrings and glutes more. This combination exercise targets the entire complex of the legs in one set.

All you need for this one is a dumbbell and a bar to grab on to (I recommend something about chest height). I'm doing this one in the rack, with a bar set on the rails. You can also use a Smith machine bar or any other solid object that you can hold on to.

I'm also using a Step platform to get a bit more range of motion on the exercises. Elevating the feet means the dumbbell doesn't hit the ground as soon when doing the squat and the knee doesn't hit the ground as soon in the lunge. It really increases the demands on the exercise.

I'm also using two dumbbells so I don't have to move a single dumbbell around.

First, grab onto the bar with an overhand grip. This is an easier way to get started, especially if you're on a Step platform.

Stand up and turn your other hand around to grip underhanded.

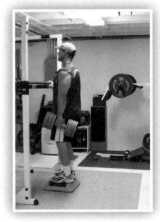

Now squat down. Keep your torso vertical and go down as far as you can.

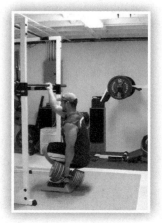

Come back up and get ready for the step-back lunge.

Step back with the left leg and the right leg will stay forward (and will be the working leg). The dumbbell will be on the outside of the left leg.

Come all the way down into the lunge position, touching the knee to the ground.

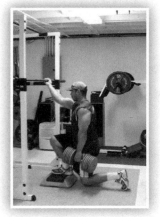

Then push back up to the standing position.

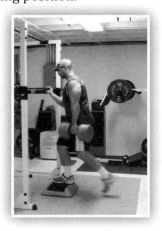

Repeat for six reps or so just working the left leg, then switch over and work the right leg. Because you're doing a squat between each lunge rep, both legs are getting pretty well worked.

The execution is the same on the other side.

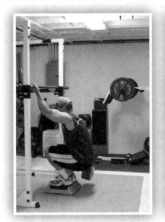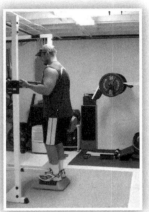

Again, I'm working with the back leg on the same side as the dumbbell.

You can also switch things up and do the step-back lunge with the dumbbell on the same side as the front leg, e.g. dumbbell in left hand, left leg stays forward.

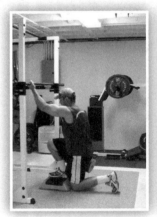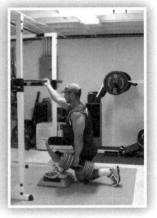

ONE-LEGGED PARTIAL SQUATS

This exercise is one I originally took to using due to a lack of enough weight plates at a gym I was going to. That and I had a bad habit of bending bars when doing regular partial squats (something to note: don't go beyond six plates on a basic silver chrome Olympic bar, like you find in most gyms)! So to get around these hurdles, I turned to the One-Legged Partial Squat.

This version is also a good one for hitting the thighs hard with very heavy weight while not totally overloading the entire body like you do with a full-on partial squat with piles of weight. You can still use a lot, but it doesn't bear down on you quite as much as a fully loaded regular top-range partial.

Also, because you're using less weight than with the full partial squat, it doesn't take as long to set up and take down, which is nice.

Using this exercise and using this very heavy amount of weight is great for training connective tissue and conditioning the muscles to much greater weights. It'll really help bring up your other lifts. Plus, it's fun to pile on so much weight that people stop and stare when they walk by the rack. :)

Instead of setting yourself up like a regular squat and doing only the top few inches, you're instead going to position yourself so that you're standing (and pushing) with only one leg.

The position of your NON-working leg is critical for balance, though. Because we not only want to maximize the amount of weight you can use with the one-legged squat, we want to maximize the safety.

So rather than just standing on one foot and squatting up and down, you will instead set the other leg directly out to the side and set it down lightly for balance. It's like an outrigger on a Hawaiian canoe. It doesn't do the work but it helps increase your center of balance so you work more effectively.

Here's the setup, done in the power rack for safety purposes. Set the safety rails to just below lockout on a regular squat. We're only looking for a few inches of range of motion with this one.

This short range of motion will maximize the power of the exercise. In this sample, I'm using six plates on either side. The first time you do this exercise, start with approximately your regular full range one Rep Max. You'll be able to go up quite a lot from there but the smaller weight will help you learn the movement to start with.

I'm also using one of the greatest weight training accessories you'll EVER see: the Manta Ray. This is a plastic molded device that snaps onto the bar. It helps distribute the weight of the bar more evenly on your back. This thing is AMAZING for squats and I consider it a necessity for heavy partials if you really want to maximize the amount of weight and therefore the benefit of the exercise.

So you're in front of the bar and ready to get started. Foot position is the key here. Your working leg should be DIRECTLY underneath the center of weight of the bar. You want a direct vertical push on that one leg. Your working leg should be slightly bent at this point.

Your OTHER leg should be out to the side and pretty much straight. I have my non-working leg actually on the frame of the rack. This helps me from cheating and helping with it because you really can't push with it up like that. It works like a charm for balance, though.

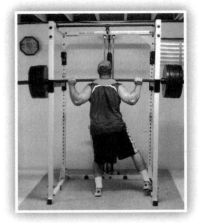

Now just straighten your working leg! Simple as that! It's a VERY short range of motion, just the top couple of inches.

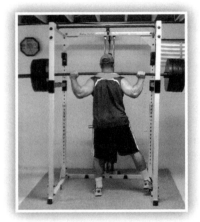

Once you've done your reps on one leg—I recommend sets of about six to ten reps on each leg—switch to the other leg.

The same setup applies: working leg directly under the center of weight of the bar and other leg out to the side.

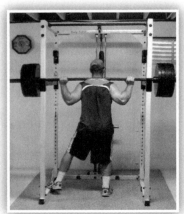

Straighten your leg and repeat!

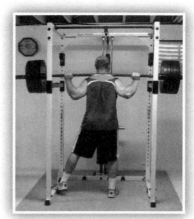

If you don't have a Manta Ray, a barbell pad or rolled up towel can help to some extent. You just need to watch out for the tendency of the bar to roll when you use the pad or towel. That's another reason why I like the Manta Ray so much. If your gym has one, perfect! If it doesn't, it's well worth the forty bucks to get one for yourself.

So give this exercise a try on your next leg workout. If you don't have a rack, you can do this one on the Smith Machine as well. I don't recommend the Smith for full range squats but they're fine for short partials like these. In fact, the Smith machine was originally designed with partial training in mind!

With the Smith machine, you can actually take your non-working foot completely off the ground, since the machine itself will balance you.

STAGGERED STEP SQUATS

T his one is just awesome for legs, I have to say. It's a barbell squat done with ONE foot up on a Step riser (or weight plate or whatever other solid object you can use to elevate one foot).

The idea with this one is to allow you to good VERY deep on one side at a time. It's tough to drop down into a fully deep squat with both legs; balance and flexibility can be an issue. But with this one, when you elevate one foot, you get extra range of motion on that elevated foot while being able to maintain good body position for the duration of the squat.

It also tends to focus more resistance on that one leg, even though you're pushing with both; the elevated leg is bent more, giving it weaker leverage, which demands more of it. So it's ALMOST like doing a one-legged squat but using two legs and without the balance requirement.

The main benefit, though, is the ability to down VERY deep on that one side without the same issues you would face going deep on a regular barbell squat.

The setup is simple: it's exactly the same as a regular squat only you set a Step platform in the rack. Just one is fine; you only need to elevate your foot a few inches. You can also try it with a barbell plate (not stacked; it's too slippery to stack one plate on top of another). A wooden block or other solid object is perfect.

Get the bar on your back, step back with your feet in close together, and then set one foot on the platform. Your feet should be a bit outside shoulder width for stability with toes pointed out somewhat.

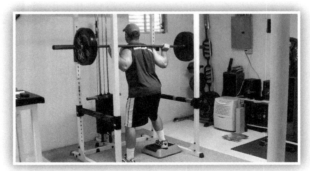

Now squat.

The key here is that you want to maintain the bar in a horizontal position during the movement, not tilted even though one leg is higher. It's that higher leg position that's going to put the stretch on the muscles of the higher side.

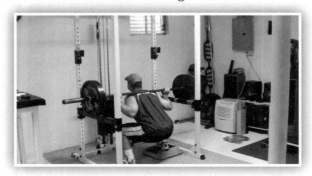

The squat itself should be done exactly like a normal squat. Take a moment at the bottom to get a good stretch, if you like. I found that to be really beneficial. Having one knee less bent means it'll have better leverage and it'll be easier to get out of the bottom than a "normal" very deep squat.

Do all your reps on one side, and rest. Then, move it over to the other side and do the same thing. I wouldn't recommend going directly over to the other side after one rep because really, both legs are getting worked no matter which side it's on. By going immediately to the other side, you'll just compromise the work you get on the second side.

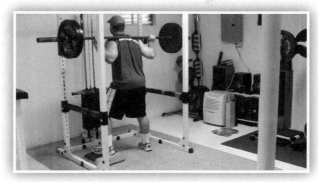

Go down into the squat and back up, keeping the bar level.

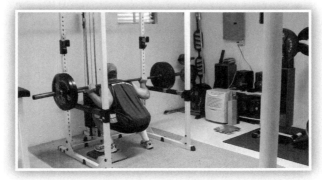

Make sure you use a weight you KNOW you can handle for a deep squat even without the Step platform, especially the first time you do it. This type of uneven staggered height is a very different feeling on the legs, hips and core.

It is a GREAT movement, though. I was really impressed with how well it hit just about everything in the lower body; it's actually the first time I've gotten sore hamstrings from squatting! Really involving the hams with a squat is tough to do and this setup seemed to make it happen, so it's definitely one I'll be including in my regular training more frequently.

TWO BARBELL HACK SQUAT "MACHINE"

I put the word "machine" in quotes because while this is actually a machine (a simple one), it's not a machine in the normal sense of the word.

This is a squat exercise setup that has some distinct advantages over the regular barbell squat.

First, it stabilizes the movement to some degree, which makes it an easier squat variation to learn. And the good thing about this stabilization is that it's not complete stabilization; because of the setup, you're only stabilizing in one plane of movement (you'll see why when you see the setup). Your body is free to find it's own path in all the other planes of movement.

Secondly, it places the hands in front of you in a neutral grip, which is much easier on the shoulders than the normal squat grip. In that respect, the grip is similar to the Safety Squat Bar, if you've seen one of those.

Naturally, the regular barbell squat is a better overall exercise and mass builder but this is a nice, targeted leg exercise that can be used instead of the squat if you can't do a normal squat for shoulder, flexibility or balance reasons.

Here's the setup:

Using a power rack, set one safety rail about four feet off the ground and the other about three feet off the ground. Set two barbells on the rails and load the top ends with a 45-pound weight plate on each one, to counterbalance what you'll be loading on the bottom.

Use 25-pound plates (or smaller) on the bottom end so that you'll be able to keep the bars close enough to each other to get them onto your shoulders. The rail height may require some adjustments to get the right height for you to get into position and get a good range of motion in the exercise. Don't worry if you don't get it perfect the first time. Just start with a light weight until you've made the adjustments.

Now, squat in front of the low ends of the bars and get your shoulders back and against the plates, with the bar ends resting on your shoulders.

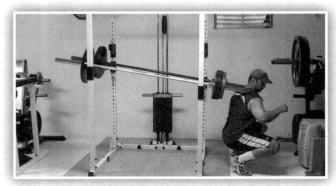

Grasp the ends of the bars and lower into the bottom squat position.

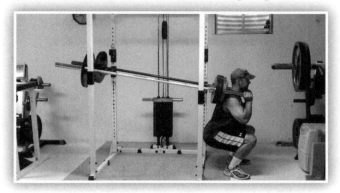

Now stand up.

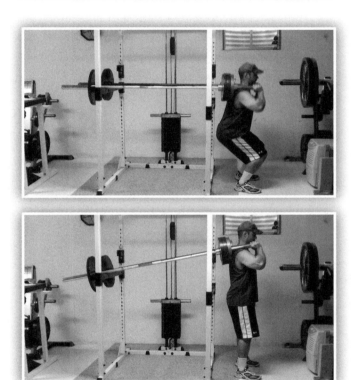

Once you're at the top, you can adjust your foot position if you need to, based on how the movement felt. Then do another rep.

With this one, you can do it two ways: continuously or resting the bars on the rail at the bottom of each rep and starting from a dead stop. The dead stop method will build power out of the bottom of a regular squat. The nice thing about that method is that it also standardizes your squat depth—you go to the rail every time.

One thing to be careful of with this one is with the barbells on the top rail, if your rack has smooth, slippery rails, the bars could slide backwards if you lean back into the movement. If that's the case for your rack, raise the top rail up higher.

Overall though, this is a nice alternative to the barbell squat.

SHOULDERS

ANGLED BAR PIKE PUSH-UPS

This is a simple variation of the pike handstand push-up done using a regular Olympic bar set on an angle. The pike push-up is a great bodyweight shoulder exercise. It's a lead-up to the regular handstand push-up, which is the king of shoulder exercises, in my opinion.

The normal version is done with your feet on a bench and your hands on the ground, body bent in a pike position (90 degrees at the waist). This version sets your hands on a bar set on an angle of about 20 to 30 degrees.

What this does is change up the angle at the shoulder, along with putting more tension on one shoulder over the other. It's a unique challenge to the entire upper body!

To do this one, you'll just need a bench or chair, a bar and something to set that bar on that is about two feet off the ground (and solid!).

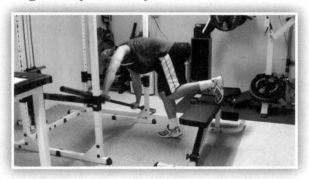

Set your feet on the bench and your hands on the bar, at about the same grip width you'd use for shoulder pressing.

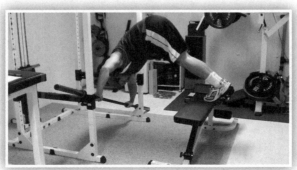

Lower yourself down, then push back up using shoulder power.

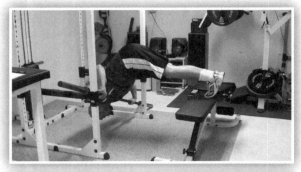

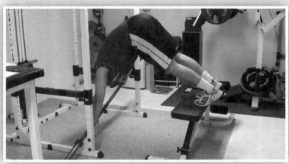

As you can see, one of the other benefits of this exercise is that it elevates your body so that your head doesn't stop the movement when it hits the ground. With the body elevated on the bar, you get a more full range of motion.

When you finish on one side, move the bench to the other side and go again, or just start your next set from that side after you rest.

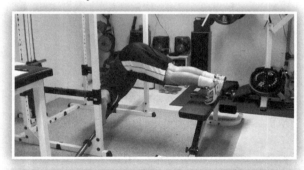

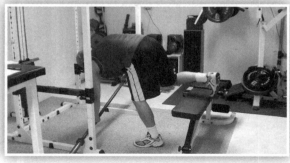

This is an excellent exercise for the shoulders and is another good "in between" exercise for those who aren't ready for a full-on handstand push-up but want some challenging bodyweight shoulder training.

NICK NILSSON

CABLE PIKE HANDSTAND PUSH-UPS

T his exercise is a killer one for the shoulders. You're going to combine a bodyweight shoulder movement with cable resistance pulling outwards. It really increases the tension on the deltoids while doing the pike handstand push-up.

This is along the same lines as the regular push-up/chest version of the exercise: Low Pulley Push-Ups, only it's done for shoulders using a shoulder-focused push-up.

So first, set a fairly light weight on the two cable stacks (this can be done with two bands as well, as long as you can tie them out wide enough to get tension) and hook on two single handles.

Set a bench a few feet back from the midline between the pulleys. Kneel down and reach over and grab the left pulley.

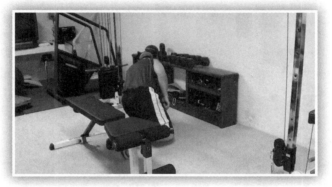

Then reach over and grab the right pulley.

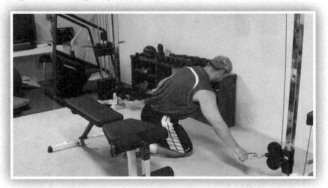

Bring your hands in towards the middle and set your fists on the floor about two feet apart.

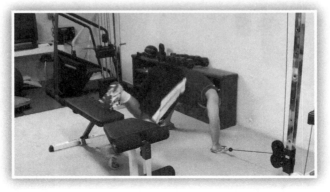

Set your feet on the bench and get your body into the pike position: legs straight, torso straight, bending only at the waist. This is essentially an easier version of the handstand push-up.

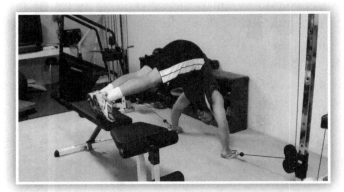

As you can see, the cables are now pulling your hands outward. It's up to you (and your delts) to prevent that from happening by actively contracting through the ENTIRE exercise.

Now lower yourself down and touch your head to the ground. Then push back up.

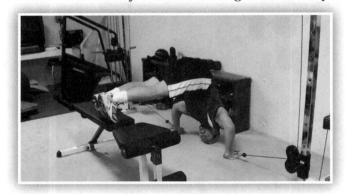

You're not doing anything ACTIVE with the pulleys; they're just there to try to pull your hands out to the sides so you have to use shoulders to prevent them from doing that. It adds an additional dimension of tension to the exercise. It is tough and effective and killer for your shoulders!

EZ BAR LEVERAGE LATERAL RAISES

The Lateral Raise is a pretty simple and pretty common exercise for the shoulders. Personally, I rarely do lateral raises, preferring to stick with presses of various forms.

There are times when I will do a few sets of laterals, just for a break from presses or to shake things up a bit. This is a great version I came up with that I've found to be really valuable.

To do this one, you'll need an EZ bar. Load ONE end. I'm using a 10-pound plate.

Grip the bar in the center with the rest of the bar tucked underneath your arm. The end will be sort-of braced against your armpit and shoulder blade.

You're going to be using the length of the bar to basically extend the levers of your arms (the bones). This is like adding weight to the end of your arm, only a bit further out to increase the leverage, making it tougher to lift your arm. It's almost as though the EZ bar becomes an extension of your arm.

Hold the bar with the plate end down, then bring it in front of your body. I like to get a bit of a swing at the start with this one because it gives a bit of a pre-stretch on the shoulders (which is something you can't get with a dumbbell lateral).

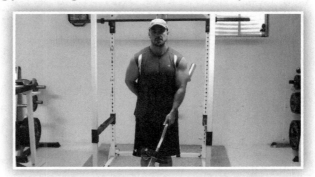

Now start bringing the bar up and to the side using lateral delt power.

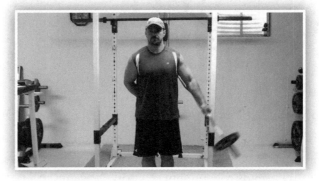

Come up as high as you can.

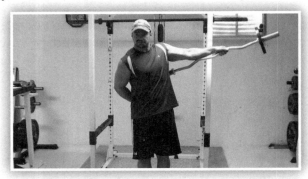

Do your reps on one side, then switch to the other. This back view will give you an idea of how the bar end gets braced behind your shoulder to maintain the bar as a lever/extension of your arm.

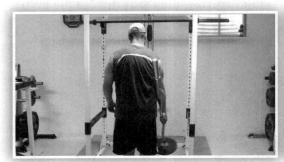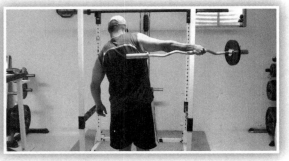

One of the benefits of this technique is that if you have a tendency to use body dipping or shrugging to get weights up, it'll self-correct immediately. This is what will happen:

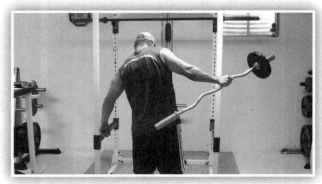

The bar will jump off your back and you won't be able to perform the movement.

So if keeping tight form is something you need to work on, this is a good option for you.

I also find that using the leverage concept is easier on the shoulder joints when I'm doing lateral raises because it spreads the tension out down the entire length of your arm rather than focusing it just on your shoulder joint.

FRONT DELTOID "PUSHOVERS" ON THE LEG CURL MACHINE

O n occasion, I think it is very useful to work the front delts in isolation (even though they get a lot of work with most pressing movements), especially if you're coming off a heavy pressing cycle and want to work more isolation stuff and back off on the weight while still getting muscle stimulation.

Also, the front delts do contribute greatly to most pressing movements; if they ARE the weak link, some extra training volume directly targeted at them is potentially beneficial.

This front delt exercise is also unique among front delt exercises. It's not completely an isolation exercise, even though it's not technically a compound exercise either.

I call it a "pushover" because it's essentially the direct opposite movement to a pullover (machine, barbell or dumbbell). It's done on the leg curl machine, which is actually perfectly suited to this exercise (if your leg curl has a lever arm in the center, you'll need to do it one arm at a time).

I'll explain it as I show you what it looks like.

First, set the ankle pads as far down as you can and put a light weight on the stack.

Sit on the floor with your back against the thigh pad of the machine and set your hands on the ankle pad like you are about to do a close-grip press.

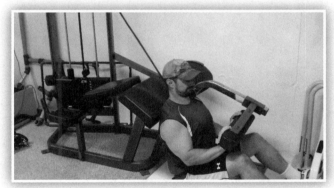

Now, using shoulder and triceps power, push the ankle pad up and around. Even though you're actively pushing with your triceps, the elbows are basically locked in place and don't actually move; they contract isometrically, allowing the front delts to take over the movement.

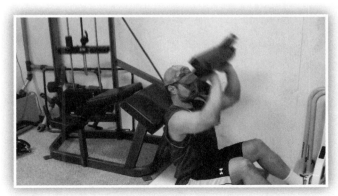

So in that respect, it's a compound exercise in which the second joint doesn't move. Come all the way up as high as you can.

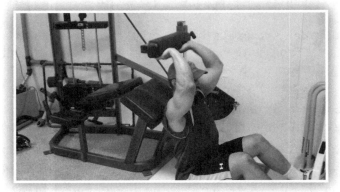

Lower the pad and you can either do the next rep without letting the stack rest or you can let it rest to regroup for the next rep (which is how I did it).

I think this technique shows good potential for improving pressing strength, much more so than a front delt raise done in isolation. Because the triceps are involved with this movement, I think there is some carryover; you'll definitely feel it in the front delts, too. I like these much better than any form of front raise I've ever tried.

JAVELIN SHOULDER PRESS

This is an excellent exercise for hitting the lateral head of the deltoids with a pressing movement. The positioning of the bar puts your hand in a neutral position, which targets that area well.

The name of the exercise comes from what it looks like as you hold it: a javelin thrower!

Of course, instead of actually throwing the barbell, you'll press it directly up (at least, if you want to keep your gym membership, you will...)

It's pretty straightforward to execute. I'm actually using a short "fat bar" (that's basically a thicker bar) in the demo here for lighter weight and higher reps. You can do this with a long Olympic bar or with an EZ curl bar as well.

The longer the bar, the trickier the balance will be on it. I also found the shorter bar to be easier to get into position for the exercise. I just picked it up in the center with my working hand and helped with the other hand, then just brought it up and around.

With a longer bar, you CAN use the same technique, just watch out for the ceiling. So in the bottom position, the bar is directly beside you, your palm facing in.

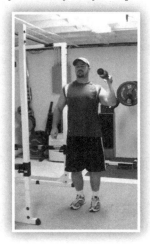

Then just press up.

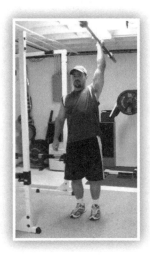

Do all your reps on one side, then repeat on the other.

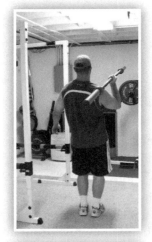

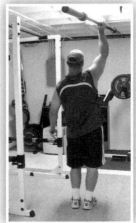

As I mentioned, I've got a pretty light weight on here since I was going for high reps. You can definitely increase the weight and reduce the reps.

ONE-ARM BARBELL HANG CLEANS
AND HANG CLEAN & PRESS

The Barbell Hang Clean and the Hang Clean & Press are two excellent upper back and shoulder exercises (even though it may sound like laundry).

The Hang Clean is essentially holding a barbell at arm's length in front of you, then using a hip thrust and powerful upper body pull to move the bar straight up, and then "rack" it across your shoulders.

The Hang Clean & Press is an extension of that movement that includes a press after the clean. THIS version is the same basic movement pattern, done with one arm instead of two.

This will obviously change up the exercise to some degree, even though it is the same basic idea. It's going to put uneven tension on the core as well as put a unique stimulus on the lower back and posterior chain during the clean.

It's going to require more balance and co-ordination and a few form tweaks to enable good execution of the exercise.

I find this to be an excellent movement for targeting the shoulders, especially with the press included. By using just one arm, it produces a unique movement pattern that hits the side delts nicely.

It's not a big mass movement, though, since you'll need to use lighter weights to compensate for the balance requirements.

It is, however, a great challenge and a lot of fun!

Ideally, you should be familiar with the regular two-arm version of both exercises before trying the one-arm version. It'll help a lot with the mechanics of the movement.

I'll start with the clean; the press is the easy part.

I'm using an Olympic bar with 10 pounds on either side. Like I said, you don't need a lot of weight. In fact, the first time you do it, start with just the bar.

Grip the bar right in the center.

Now stand up with the bar hanging at arm's length in front of you.

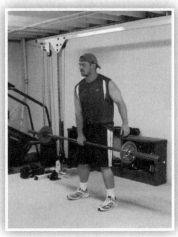

Here's the trick with the clean: lean forward like you're doing the top part of a stiff-legged deadlift. The real power for this exercise comes from the hip thrust movement (like a kettlebell swing).

Shift your butt back, and then when you're ready to do the clean, explosively thrust your hips forward. This pulls the upper body back very quickly, which translates the power to the arm. This transfer of power means you're not pulling primarily with the arm, you're generating power through the hips.

It's a point about cleans that a lot of people miss: it isn't an arm exercise even though the arms are involved.

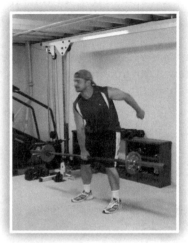

So explode the hips forward, pulling the bar up fast.

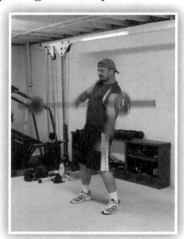

As the bar gets close to your shoulders, flip your wrist back to "rack" the bar across your shoulders.

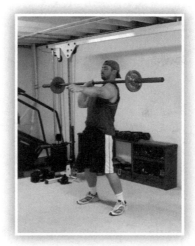

The key with the one-arm version is that you need to bring your non-working arm up and hold it straight out in front of you to help stabilize the bar in the rack position.

Don't try and just hold it with one arm across your upper chest; it doesn't work well if your other arm is not in position, too. If your other arm is at your side, the shoulder girdle tilts forward, which makes it tougher to hold that position.

To get the bar back down, just flip the barbell forward again and return it to the hanging position. That's the easy part.

You can do just the One-Arm Barbell Clean as an exercise in its own right and it's very effective.

We're also going to add the Press part here (I'll shows pictures with the left arm doing the full sequence this time). Here's the dead hang to start:

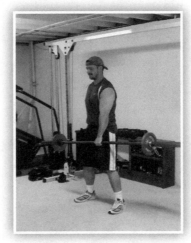

Now the bend forward, sticking the butt out to wind up for the hip thrust.

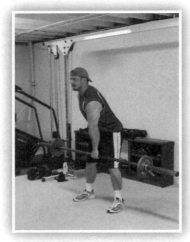

Now the explosive hip thrust forward and the powerful pull up on the bar.

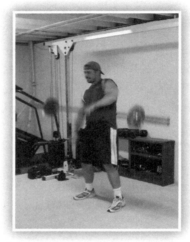

Flip the wrist as you come to the top and bring the non-working side arm up to help rack the bar.

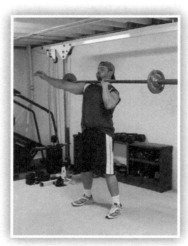

Now press the bar to lockout.

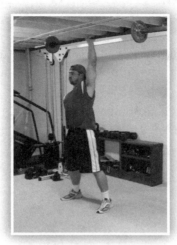

The press requires balance and good shoulder strength since you'll be starting from that complete bottom-start position. Grip the bar hard; you'll need to use your grip to keep the bar balanced overhead.

Lower the bar back down to your shoulder, then flip it back down and hang at arm's length.

Those are the two basic variations. Again, start with just the bar the first time you do these. They take some practice since they're not just straight up-and-down movements like a lot of bodybuilding exercises.

ONE DUMBBELL SHOULDER PRESS
GOBLET STYLE

This version of the shoulder press resembles a "strongman" type of movement in which you're treating the dumbbell like an oddly-shaped object rather than a dumbbell.

It a front-delt-accentuated exercise, similar to an Arnold Press, but without rotating the elbows around because they're set on the dumbbell (you'll see what I mean).

First, you'll need a moderate to heavy dumbbell (just one). Set it on the floor. Reach down and grab it with both hands.

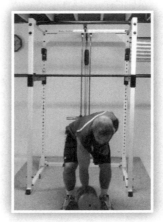

Lift the dumbbell to your chest and lean back so you're supporting the dumbbell on your chest.

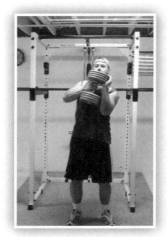

Now change your grip from on the handle to putting your palms under the dumbbell plates so that your fingers are gripping the sides of the plates. The dumbbell is being held vertically.

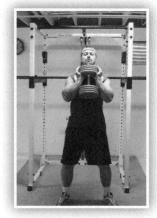

Press directly up as high as you can.

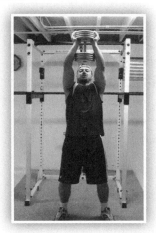

Lower down, then press again. Simple from there—it's just a straight-up shoulder press using a different way of holding the dumbbell.

When you're done with the set, lean back and rest it on your chest again. Grab the handles and set it back down on the ground.

This is a nice change of pace from regular shoulder pressing. The closer grip hits the front delts nicely.

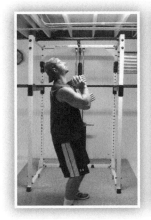 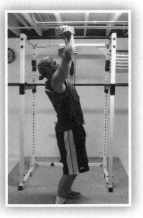

REAR DELT IN-SET SUPERSET:
SHOULDER PRESS TO PULL-UPS

R ear delts make for a complete physique. Unfortunately, the rear delts can be a tough muscle to hit; bent-over lateral raises will hit them well in isolation and are useful to some degree. But, to really BUILD muscles, you need to use compound exercises.

Here's the problem: there ARE no compound exercises that specifically target the rear delts. Shoulder presses utilize the rear delts to help stabilize the shoulder joint, not to actually press the weight up.

The rear delts function to pull the humerus (the upper arm bone) posteriorly (to the back), not to raise it up in a vertical movement pattern—that's the front and side delts at work, along with the triceps.

Rowing and pull-up movements actually give you a more direct attack on the rear delts according to their actual function, but the large powerful muscles of the back (like the lats, teres major and rhomboids) tend to take over, leaving the rear delts out in the cold.

That's where THIS exercise combination comes in. You're going to work two directly antagonistic exercises that each hit the rear delts. It's basically the only common denominator between the two compound exercises.

And yes, that means this combination is going to BLAST your rear delts extremely hard; everything else gets a rest at some point between the two exercises. The rear delts get ZERO rest.

This combination is done in what I like to call an "In-Set Superset." What that means is instead of doing a normal superset with a full set of one exercise and then immediately doing a full set of the other exercise, you're going to alternate reps of each exercise, and these exercises must share a common position so that you can transition smoothly between the two with no break.

You'll see exactly what I'm talking about once I show you the exercise in action here.

You're going to be doing a kneeling barbell shoulder press alternated with a leg-assisted pull-up, both done using the same barbell.

This one is best done in the power rack. Kneel in the rack and set the safety rails to just below shoulder height.

Set the racking hooks about two feet higher. Try this with just the bar as a dry run so you get the heights right before you add weight.

Start with the bar on the rails next to the uprights of the rack and kneel down. Grab the bar with a moderate to wide grip. I usually use a grip a bit inside my bench press grip for shoulder press.

Get the bar into the start position for the shoulder press (I'll give you the back and side views side-by-side here).

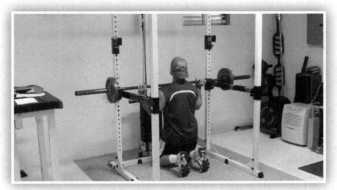

As you press up it's CRITICAL that you push your head forward under the bar. This is what activates the rear delts (albeit to stabilize the shoulder joint). Force those elbows back and get your head under the bar.

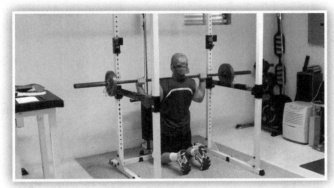

Once you've hit lockout, move the bar forward until it hits the uprights of the rack, and then set it down into the racking hooks. This is where you'll need to make any adjustments to the height of those hooks—you don't want it to be a stretch to get the bar up and in and but you also don't want them to be too low that you end up dropping the bar more than a few inches into them.

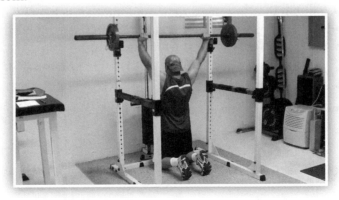

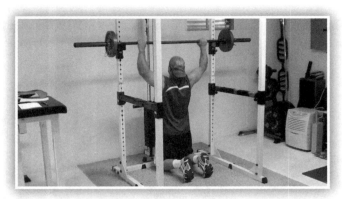

Now do the pull-up. Keep your toes on the ground and use your legs to guide and assist the movement so that you can use EXTREMELY strict form, pulling your elbows back as far as you can and pulling yourself up until the bar hits your upper chest.

This is VERY important as the higher you pull and the more you can focus on pulling your elbows back, the harder the rear delts will be worked.

The toes on the ground are important to achieving that maximum range of motion and for taking up some of your bodyweight. If you get your feet off the ground, your bodyweight will result in the bigger muscles of the back kicking in too much, defeating the purpose of the exercise. Your toes on the ground also allows you to push your body forward as you pull your elbows back.

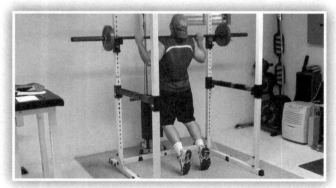

Lower yourself back down to your knees, get the bar off the racking hooks, and then lower back to the bottom of the shoulder press position. Don't set the bar back down on the rails; keep it at shoulder level when you start the next rep.

Repeat until your rear delts are basically screaming. They will be the continuous link between these two exercises and will get worked HARD.

You'll feel them when you finish the set and you will likely feel them like you never have before.

This is a GREAT rear delt exercise that utilizes two compound movements to push that smaller muscle they have in common to the limit.

NICK NILSSON

SIDE-TO-SIDE BARBELL SHOULDER PRESSES

I f you're like me, shoulders are one of the toughest body parts to develop. So I've had to develop effective ways to really hit my shoulders HARD and get the best results possible.

This exercise is one of my favorites for building strength and explosive power in the shoulders. I've found it to be <u>VERY</u> effective for hitting the lateral delts as well, which is critical for building shoulder width.

To perform this exercise, you'll need a barbell and a power rack. That's it!

Instead of pressing the barbell from inside the rack, though, and taking a traditional grip on the bar, you will be standing OUTSIDE the rack on one side, facing in. You'll be pressing ONE END of the bar, using the other end as a pivot point.

First, you'll need to set one of the safety rails up near the top of the rack—about forehead level is good. The other rail should be set at just about shoulder height.

Set an Olympic barbell across these rails so that it's sloping down to one side. Load the high end of the barbell with at least one weight plate (45 or 35 pounds) to counterbalance the end you'll be pressing.

Load the lower end of the bar with weight. Start with a weight that is fairly light (if you can do dumbbell presses with 50-pound dumbbells, start with just a 45-pound plate on the bar) until you get an idea of how the exercise works. THEN you can start adding plates. Also, **be VERY sure you've got good collars on BOTH ends of the bar**—you don't want any plates sliding off.

Now you're ready to start the exercise.

Stand at the low end of the bar (outside the rack) facing in towards the rack. Grip the end of the bar with both hands (not overlapping but butted up so they're right BESIDE each other on the end of the bar). One will be closer to the end than the other. You can switch that grip on the next set to keep things even.

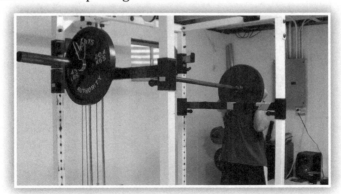

Note how the left side rail is up near the top (about forehead height), and the working side rail is at about shoulder level. Standing on the outside of the rack facing in towards the barbell, take a staggered grip on the very end of the bar.

Stand a little off to one side to start with. When you do the exercise, you're basically going to be doing a press with one hand (using the other hand for guidance and balance), bringing the bar up and overhead, and then lowering it down on the other side. Then you'll repeat, going back over to the other side.

The press comes primarily from the left arm here. The right arm is just for guidance and balance.

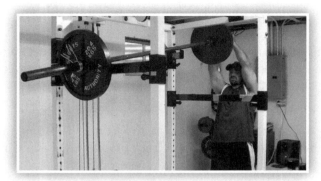

Now it's a press to the top. Once you're at the top, start lowering the end of the bar down to the other side, taking up the weight on your right arm.

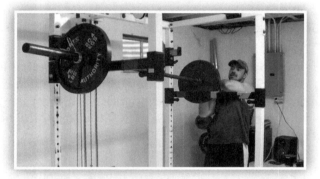

Now the weight is all on the right arm with the left arm for balance.

Here's a side view of the exercise. Note the staggered grip on the end of the bar. One hand is right at the end, and the other hand is on the bar pressed right against the first hand but NOT on top of it.

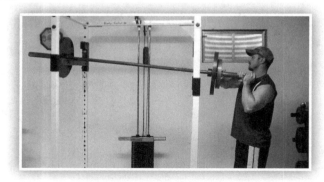

Here's the press to the top.

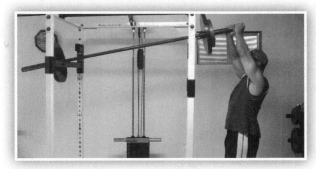

Then down on the other side.

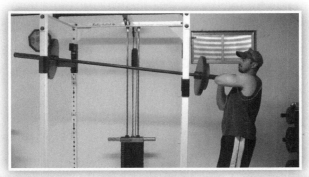

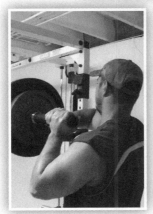 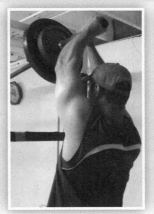 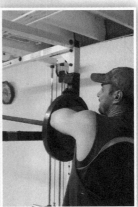

You can see why I call it the "Side-To-Side Shoulder Press." You start with, for example, a left-hand one-arm press, bringing the bar overhead and across, and then perform a right-handed one-arm press. You go back and forth until you've done as many reps as you can.

When you're doing the press (especially at the bottom of the movement), be careful to use the other hand primarily for guidance and balance, NOT to try and pull up on the bar for help. That other shoulder will be in an awkward position to exert force and you don't want to risk injury.

If you want to REALLY finish off the shoulders (I like to do this on my last set), when you're done with the side-to-side movement you can continue with a two-arm press directly to the front.

 CR   CR   CR

Overall, this exercise is an excellent alternative to barbell and dumbbell presses. It's a novel yet EXTREMELY

functional shoulder exercise that has the potential to build excellent power and strength in the shoulders.

The positioning of the bar, the side-to-side movement and the fact that you're gripping a MUCH thicker portion of the bar each contributes to the overall effectiveness of the exercise.

I think you're going to like it!

TOWEL PLATE LATERAL RAISES

I love exercises that use equipment not only in ways you've never thought they could be used in but exercises that make equipment out of things you never really even thought WERE equipment!

That's the beauty of this exercise; it's a lateral raise done with a towel and a weight plate. You're going to string a towel (at least two to three feet long, ideally) through the center hole of a weight plate (I'm using a 25-pound plate).

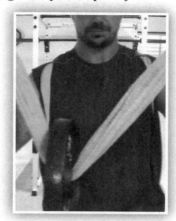

Then you're going to grip the ends, with the plate hanging down in front of you.

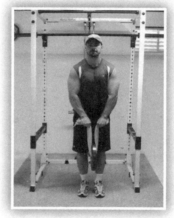

Now you're going to do a lateral raise, bringing your hands up and out to the sides as you raise the plate up. The cool thing is, because you're also straightening out the towel, you're getting direct sideways resistance on the side delts, which is VERY effective on those side delts.

This is my preferred way to do lateral raises, to be honest. Once you've tried it, you won't want to go back to regular raises.

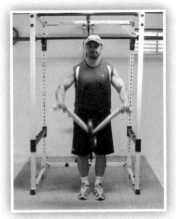

Go up until the plate is at your upper chest and hold for a moment, if you can. The plate will come in contact with your upper chest. Your upper arms should be almost horizontal and your forearms will be up a bit higher.

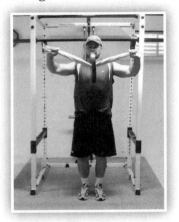

Lower and repeat. Here's a side view.

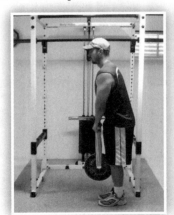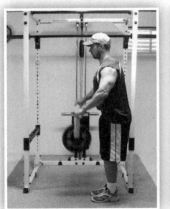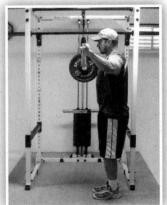

This is a really simple way to essentially double the effective tension on the side delts when performing a lateral raise. You get the up-and-down resistance of gravity and the lateral resistance from the effort of straightening out the towel.

TRICEPS

BAND SUPPORTED DIPS

Let me just start by saying, even if you're STRONG at doing dips, this exercise is going to challenge you like you're never been challenged by a dip before.

To give you an idea, I can do 50 reps of bodyweight dips, but five reps with this version is tough.

But don't let that scare you! You're going to LOVE this one. This is GREAT exercise for the entire upper body. Basically, instead of using bars for dipping, you're going to throw a couple of bands over a couple of bars and use THOSE for dipping. The setup requires a rack, but it's really easy to put together.

First, of course, you'll need some bands. They'll need to be fairly thick bands because they'll be supporting your weight during the exercise.

I'm using the green bands for this exercise and they're just about perfect.

So, set the safety rails in your power rack as high up as they go, and put two Olympic bars on the rails. Next, throw a band over each bar. You're not tying the bands on, just folding them in half over top of the bars.

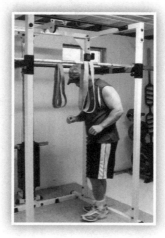

Set your hands in the band loops.

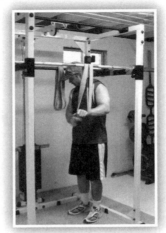

Now get yourself ready to dip:

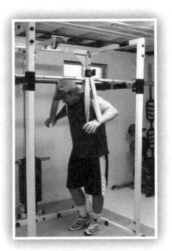

Get in the locked-out position. Here's where the fun starts...

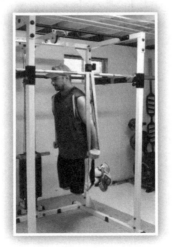

Slowly lower yourself to the bottom of the dip. Be very sure to do this slowly and under control. If you drop down quickly, your balance will be compromised. Every moment you're suspending yourself (I probably should have called this one Band Suspended Dips, come to think of it), you're entire upper body is clenched to balance.

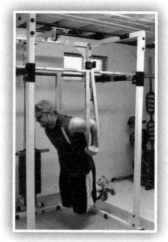

So you're in the bottom position. Now it's time to get back up.

Use a powerful push downwards to get yourself back up. Because you're using bands, you'll have to push down hard in order to stretch the bands and get enough tension to raise yourself up.

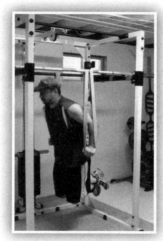

With that big push, you're going to bounce up higher than where you started. Be prepared to re-stabilize yourself when you come down from that bounce.

Keep going for as many reps as you can.

This is a tough exercise but VERY effective. Your triceps, chest and shoulders will be on fire after just a few reps.

BARBELL LEVER PUSHDOWNS

O ne of the toughest parts of having a basic home gym setup is that you don't often have access to a cable machine. This limits a lot of the things you can do; for example, pushdowns.

How do you do a pushdown without a cable machine to work with?

Easy! You utilize a simple leverage setup using a barbell and power rack. Even if you DO have a cable machine you can use, I encourage you to try this as well; I find it has a GREAT effect on the triceps because you're moving actual weight instead of cable. It works like a free-weight exercise rather than a cable exercise.

Also, since you're going to be gripping the thick end of the barbell, you'll see increased activity in the triceps (thick bars work great for mass-building).

I'm going to show you a few variations of the Barbell Lever Pushdown that will blow your triceps up fast!

Set one of the safety rails at about waist height, and set the other rail just about a foot and a half off the ground. Now load a plate onto the lower end and shift the bar over so that the end of the bar rests on the lower rail.

Here's what the setup and top position looks like:

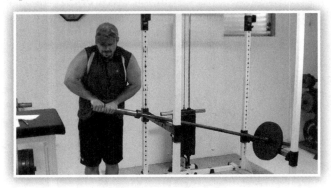

So, in that top position, stand close to the bar and set your hands on it. I have my elbows out wide to the sides on this one; if you're using a light weight, you can also set your elbows in close to your sides like a regular pushdown.

Now, push the end of the bar directly down. Simple as that!

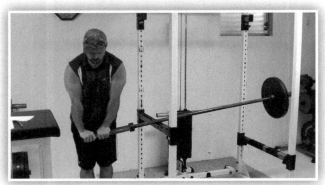

A good variation of this exercise is to stand at the end and use both hands on the end of the bar at the same time.

The difference in grip here is that your shoulders will be rotated inwards. This hits the outer triceps VERY hard—great for building thickness in the arms.

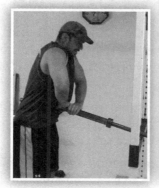 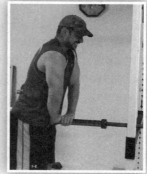

You can also change your grip on the bar to be a little bit wider, which will allow you to use more weight.

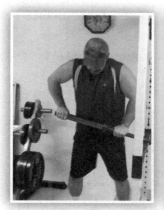 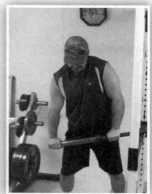

Now the final trick...

When you DO use more weight, you'll also need a way to increase your own bodyweight so that you can actually get leverage on the bar.

To do THAT, wear a dip belt loaded with a plate or two. That will instantly increase your bodyweight and give you better leverage during the exercise.

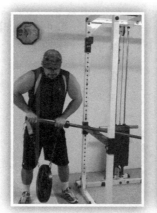 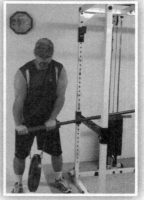

Plus, you can use the same dip belt technique with the end-position technique as well:

So if you've got access to a rack and a barbell, you're good to go! Give this pushdown lever exercise a try and feel those triceps swell!

BARBELL BODYWEIGHT TRICEPS EXTENSIONS/PULL- INS

The long head of the triceps has two functions. The first is pretty much just like the other heads of the triceps, which is to extend the elbow. The unique part about the long head is that it primarily does this when the upper arm is vertical overhead. So to really hit it with triceps work, you need to do arms-overhead stuff.

The other function of the long head is very similar to the lats: adducting the humerus, meaning it brings the upper arm in towards the body. That's why when you do some back training (like pullovers) you'll also feel it in your triceps.

This exercise targets both functions of the long head in one movement. To do this one, you'll just need a barbell and some plates (and a riser, if you want to increase your range of motion—you'll see).

First, load the plates on the bar. I recommend 45's for height. The actual weight on the bar doesn't matter, since bodyweight will be the resistance, not the bar. It's just there as a means of movement.

I like to use a Step riser so that I get a greater range of motion at the bottom and a bigger stretch. Set that behind the bar.

Kneel on the riser and set your hands on the bar about six inches or so apart.

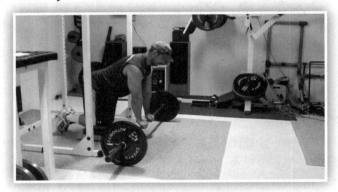

Now roll the bar forward, just like an abdominal roll-out movement. The key here to hitting the triceps is that as you go down, bend your elbows so that your forehead comes down on top of the bar (not to smack it but just touch it). The riser allows you to get a bit more stretch at the bottom by keeping your elbows off the floor just a little longer.

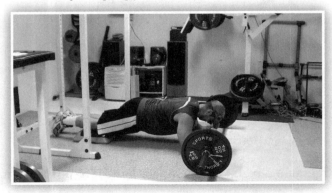

Keep your elbows in tight. This puts the stretch on the long head. It's not a fully overhead position, but it's enough to put a good stretch on the long head.

Now, using triceps power like a push-down/push-up type of movement, push your body up, and THEN start pulling the bar back in towards your legs. This is the part that works the adducting function of the long head.

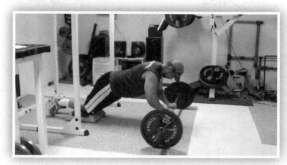

Combining these two movements is something you can't do with machines or most free weight exercises. It's a one-two punch on the long head of the triceps and, as a bonus, it will also hit your abs quite hard. The roll-out movement is one of the best exercises you can do for abs!

You can do this exercise with your knees on the floor as well. You don't need the riser, it's just there for extra range of motion.

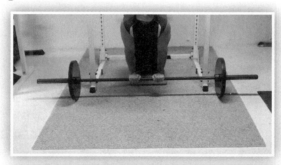

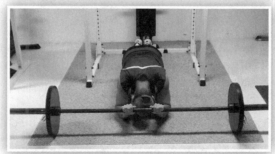

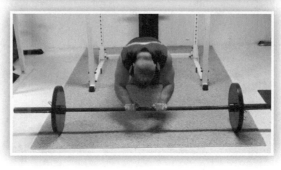

DECLINE BENCH FLARED-ELBOW TRICEPS PUSH-UPS

I have to say; this is one of THE best bodyweight triceps exercises I've ever used. It requires the use of a decline bench or slant board and your bodyweight, and that's it.

The exercise is essentially a close-grip bench press done with your hands (or fists, as I prefer it) on the lower end of the bench, and your knees on the top pads of the decline bench itself.

The decline position puts more of your bodyweight onto your triceps and the flared elbow position really targets the lateral head of the triceps, giving you wider-looking arms and a better-defined horseshoe.

So here's the setup:

Stand in front of the bench, walk your hands forward on the bench, and get your thighs and knees on the top end. I like to clench my fists and use them as the pivot rather than flat palms. I find this allows me to roll onto the edges of my hands during the movement, which actually takes stress OFF the wrists during the exercise.

You're not going to place your knuckles on the bench, though; you still want the heels of your hands on the bench. Just curl your fingers up into a fist instead of placing them flat on the bench.

Start with your elbows straight.

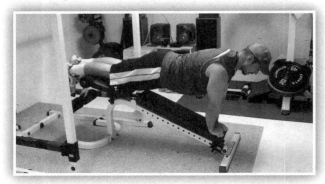

Now, lower your torso all the way down to the bench. And I do mean ALL the way; that's one of the big benefits of this exercise. Because you're up off the ground, your elbows and forearms can actually dip below the level of the bench. If you did these on the floor, the floor would stop the movement.

As you come down, your elbows should flare directly out to the sides.

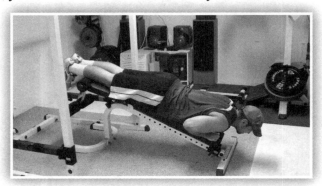

Then, push back up to the start position, squeezing the triceps hard at the top.

To make these a bit harder, you can move your knees forward on the top of the bench so that more of your bodyweight is bearing down. You can also (if you have one) wear a weighted vest (the weights in the vest will decrease your range of motion, though).

Here's a straight-on view of the exercise.

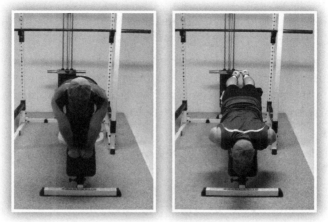

Very simple in execution and VERY effective for hitting the triceps surprisingly hard.

FEET SUSPENDED CLOSE-GRIP PUSH-UPS

I love exercises utilizing unique setups that dramatically increase the resistance used in bodyweight exercises. Basically, when you get to a certain level of strength in a bodyweight movement and can do a lot of reps with it, it isn't as effective for building more muscle and strength.

But if you can adjust your body position and make it harder, then you can keep making progress. This exercise is an example of that with the close-grip push-up.

For this specific setup, you'll need a power rack. If you don't have a power rack, you can do these with your feet up on something else solid (like a railing or countertop, for example) with your hands on the floor instead of on a bar. You don't absolutely NEED a rack to do this type of feet-suspended movement (feet not just elevated, but actually suspended is what we're looking for).

This set-up is going to force more of your bodyweight onto the triceps as you're doing the close-grip push-up exercise.

Set one bar in the rack at about shoulder height (where you'd set it for squats). Set the rails to about 2 feet off the ground or so (a little above knee height worked for me) and set another bar on those, pushed against the uprights.

Hold the lower bar in a close grip, about shoulder-width apart. Stand facing that bar with your back to the other bar, and then bring your upper body down to the bar.

Next, reach up and back with one leg to hook your toes over the bar.

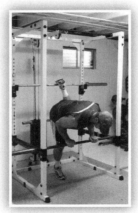

Once that's solidly hooked, bring your other leg up and hook those toes over the bar, too.

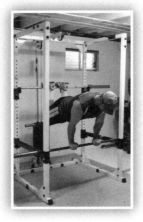

Now you're in the bottom position of the close-grip push-up on the bar.

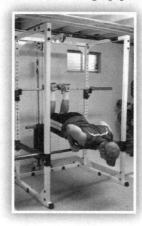

Now just do the push-up!

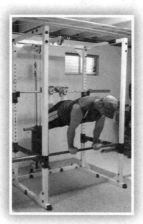

This exercise looks a lot easier than it actually is. By suspending your bodyweight in this fashion, you actually put more of your bodyweight on the triceps as resistance, more so than close-grip presses with feet elevated on a bench or something else.

If you want to get even more out of this and need more resistance, you can also do it with a weight vest on or put the bottom bar lower.

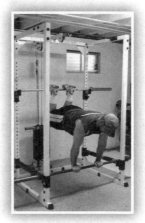

IN-SET SUPERSET OF PUSHDOWNS AND FLARED ELBOW PUSHDOWNS

This is an excellent pushdown combination exercise, covering two types in one In-Set Superset style set. An In-Set Superset is a technique in which you alternate reps of two different exercises that share a similar position; in this case, the bottom position of the pushdown.

Once you see how it's done, it's very intuitive. It's also extremely beneficial in that you work the target muscle from two different angles in one exercise. This places substantially greater demands on the muscle, which can really lead to great gains in that muscle. It's one of my favorite techniques.

Start with a normal straight-bar pushdown.

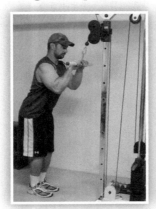 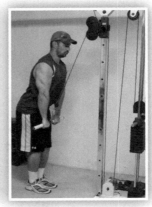

Now at the bottom position, instead of coming back up in a regular pushdown, you're going to come up in a flared-elbow pushdown, keeping the bar in close to your body.

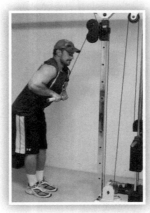 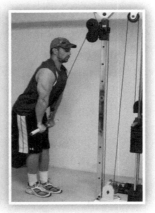

This targets the lateral head of the triceps very strongly, which is not as strongly worked with the normal pushdown form.

Now come back up in the regular pushdown, then do a regular pushdown again and repeat with alternating reps of the two variations.

When you come to that bottom position, try and push the bar down to the floor, even when your arms are already straight. This will more fully engage the long head of the triceps, which has a role in shoulder adduction.

This combination exercise will really light up your triceps well.

KNEELING CABLE NOT-KICKBACKS FOR TRICEPS

T he kickback is obviously not a big mass-building type of exercise; however, for maximizing the contraction on the triceps muscles, the peak point of the exercise is incredibly effective.

This makes the kickback a very useful tool in your training toolbox when used for the proper purpose, which is peak contraction.

THIS version of the kickback is done with the low pulley and I call it a "not-kickback" because the movement pattern, while it ends in the top kickback position, is more like a backwards press.

This allows you to use significantly more weight, which means a HUGE peak contraction at the top of the movement, much more so than normal kickbacks done with the "hinge" type of isolation movement. Think of this as a compound kickback.

For this one, you'll need a low pulley and a single handle. I also added a short length of chain to make it easier to get the weight into position. Set a fairly light weight on the pulley the first time you do it, then move up from there once you see how it's done and how it's different from the regular kickback.

Kneel in front of the low pulley and brace one hand on the floor or on the foot of the machine.

Get the cable handle in position with your hand near your hip and bend your elbow, bringing it up and behind your body.

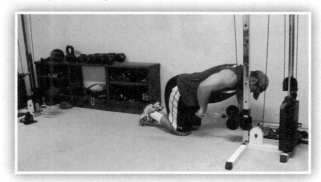

Now, since the real "money" part of this exercise is the peak contraction, we're not doing a classic full range of motion here; we're going for the max at the top.

Now start pushing backwards like you're doing a press, rather than doing a kickback.

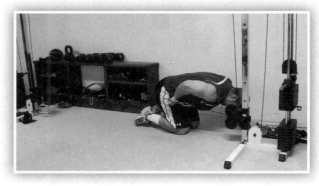

Push backwards until your arm is straight, and keep pushing backwards, moving your shoulder back as well. Try to squeeze as much contraction out as you can, and hold that squeeze for a few seconds before coming back to the start position.

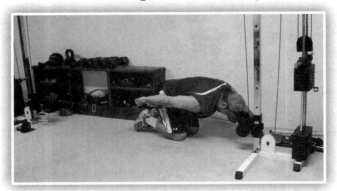

Again, the peak contraction is what we're focused on here; the rest of the exercise is just a means to get you into that maximum contracted position that is anatomically possible for the triceps, so don't sacrifice weight for range of motion. We want it moderately loaded (much more so than regular cable kickbacks) for a shorter range.

Do four to six reps on one side, then switch to the other.

This is a great exercise to finish off the triceps after you've hit them with other exercises. I wouldn't necessarily do this one on its own.

You could do decline close grip bench, then an extension type of movement, and then finish with this one and your triceps will be TOAST.

MODIFIED MUSCLE-UP FOR TRICEPS

The Muscle Up is a very cool bodyweight exercise. It's a two-part movement that basically has you doing a pull-up, and then a dip or pushdown movement to get your body up over the bar.

It's a TOUGH exercise, requiring a lot of strength and coordination (and high ceilings) but the results you can get in your back, arms and shoulders are phenomenal!

So what do you do if you either don't have the strength to do a full-on muscle-up or don't have high enough ceilings to do one either (which is my problem).

You do THIS modified version of the exercise, which takes up some of your bodyweight and lowers the height so it can be done even in a basement. And, when done using a power rack, also has the advantage of being able to roll the bar forward as you transition.

This modified version will primarily hit the triceps (you could almost call it a bodyweight pushdown). By setting the bar higher, you can do the pull-up part of it better, but you won't be able to push yourself up over the bar with your feet set on the bench (you'll see with the setup).

Here's how the setup goes: set the rails in the power rack to about the level of the bottom of your ribcage. Set a bar on top of the rails. Set a bench parallel to the bar just a few feet out from the bar.

You can adjust the bar height and bench distance once you start doing the exercise.

Set your hands on the bar about shoulder-width apart (palms down), and stand on the bench.

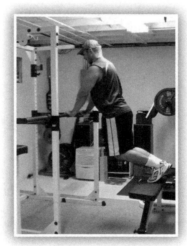

Now, keeping the core tight, lower yourself down, bending at the elbows and knees. Your arm position will look like the top of a pushdown (which is also the top of a reverse grip pull-up!). Knees should be bent with toes on the bench.

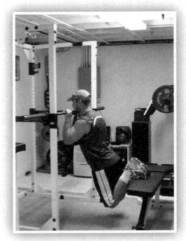

Now, using triceps power (and a little leg help, if you need it), push yourself directly up as though doing a bodyweight pushdown.

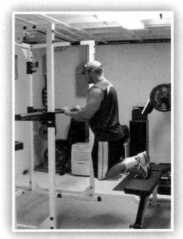

As you push yourself up, the bar will roll forward a little (which is why the rack is so useful for this). Go all the way up until your arms are fully extended and locked out.

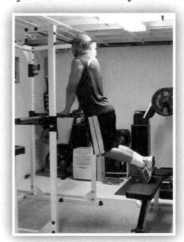

Lower yourself down, reversing the movement, and repeat.

As you can see, doing it without the bench would make it a LOT harder. Doing a "free" muscle-up requires tremendous strength in the upper body. This variation makes the benefits of the exercise a bit more accessible if you either don't have enough strength for the full movement or don't have high enough ceilings (which is what I run into with it).

ON-BARBELL TRICEPS EXTENSION-PRESSES

T his one, like the name indicates, is a combination of close grip push-up, a triceps extension and almost a horizontal pike handstand push-up or Arnold press.

For this exercise you'll need a barbell and a bench (or chair) and something to brace the barbell on. I'm using a rack but it can be anything solid.

Load a couple of plates on the bar to get it up off the ground a bit. Then, push it up against the solid object (the uprights of the rack are easiest). Set a bench a few feet back from the bar (it can parallel or lengthwise, it doesn't matter).

Set your hands on the bar about shoulder-width apart and set your feet on the bench.

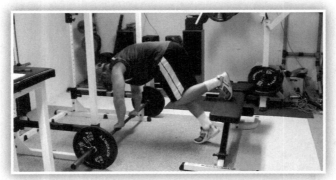

Get yourself into a pike position with your arms straight and locked out. This is the start position. This pike position is what makes it different than a standard close-grip push-up.

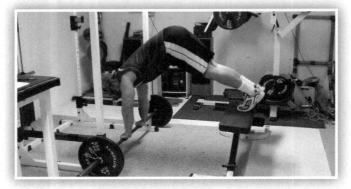

Now, lower yourself down and forward, bending your arms and straightening out the body as you do so.

Bring your body all the way down until your stomach is touching the bar. This is the bottom position.

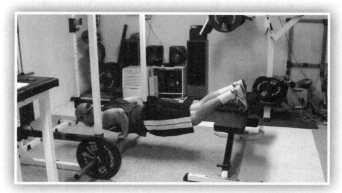

Now here comes the critical part: you're NOT just going to do a close-grip push-up here. You're going to push yourself UP and BACK into the pike position.

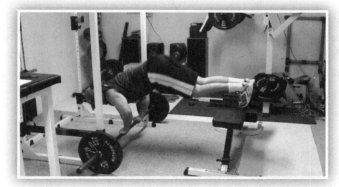

When you're at the top, be sure to push yourself all the way up and fully lock out your arms. Push your butt as high in the air as you can. This also kicks in the long head of the triceps, bringing in the extension function of the triceps.

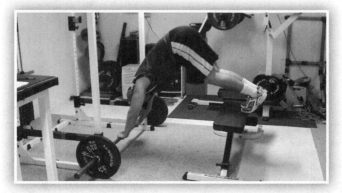

You're not only doing a close-grip press but also using them to push your body back up to the pike position. It's a nice multiple-angle, bodyweight hit to the tri's. Even if you're strong, this'll have your triceps toasted with 6 to 10 reps.

UNSTABLE BAR BODYWEIGHT
TRICEP EXTENSIONS

This is a GREAT bodyweight tricep exercise that hits the long head of the triceps, the one that is the largest and has the greatest growth potential.

As you get stronger at the exercise, I've got yet another variation of it for you here which is done on an unstable bar. And let me tell you, it's BRUTAL. Every second of every rep, as you go down and come back is spent fighting to keep your balance on the bar. It'll light up your triceps like crazy.

This is done using a pulley bar attachment. I've attached to an actual pulley set up for convenience but you can very easily loop a chain around just about anything and clip a bar onto it and achieve the same effect.

The basic idea is that instead of using a solid bar, you're using a handle that is balanced in the center. This places tremendous stabilization demands on the triceps.

It's a simple exercise to execute:

Have the bar a few feet off the ground with your feet about three feet away. The closer you set your feet to the bar, the less resistance you'll have, so start in closer first, and move out as you learn the exercise.

Set your hands on the bar, fairly close to the center balancing point.

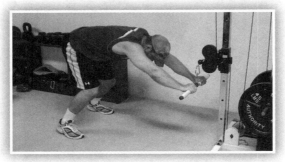

Now, bending only at the elbows, slowly lower your head down under the handle. DO NOT go fast on this one...it won't end well. This is a controlled movement in order to keep your balance on the handle.

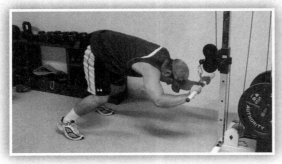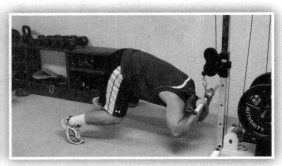

Extend back up and repeat.

By the time you're done, I can promise your triceps will be on fire. Aim for about five to seven reps or so with this one.

ABOUT THE AUTHOR

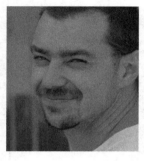

Nick Nilsson is known in the fitness world as the "Mad Scientist of Exercise," and for good reason. For more than 20 years, Nick has been creating unique, new exercises and training techniques and putting together some of the most innovative muscle-building and fat-loss programs available anywhere.

To create these unique programs and exercises, Nick puts to work his degree in Physical Education, covering advanced biomechanics, kinesiology, anatomy and physiology. When you put his exercises and programs to work, you'll immediately see and feel exactly how this combination of science, practical knowledge, thinking outside the box and just a little bit of insanity really mesh together to maximize every aspect of your training!

Nick uses his experience as a former skinny guy to help your build the body of your dreams, whether it is building muscle, losing fat or both! He has helped literally THOUSANDS of people accomplish their goals and achieve results above and beyond the reach of more traditional programs.

More Books from Nick

MUSCLE EXPLOSION: 28 DAYS TO MAXIMUM MASS

I f you are part of the conventional wisdom crowd, take a very deep breath... with **Muscle Explosion** you're going to:

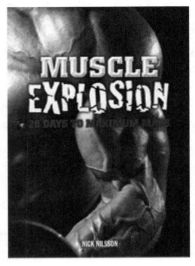

- Reduce caloric intake to well below maintenance levels and eliminate protein completely (in very specific ways for very specific purposes)
- Aim to overtrain
- Train the same body part five days in a row
- Perform the same exercise five days in a row

Muscle Explosion literally turns conventional muscle-building wisdom inside-out and upside down. By practicing the groundbreaking training and eating strategies in this book, you will SHATTER your genetic limitations by literally changing your physiology, quickly setting the stage for EXPLOSIVE increases in muscle mass and strength. Each cycle of this program lasts only 28 days and the workouts take less than an hour to complete. This book is for the intermediate to advanced trainer who is ready to DEMOLISH plateaus and achieve growth and strength increases previously thought unattainable.

MAD SCIENTIST MUSCLE: BUILD "MONSTER" MASS WITH SCIENCE-BASED TRAINING!

T hink changing your physiology is impossible? THINK AGAIN... With **Mad Scientist Muscle**, you'll use science-based training techniques, like "controlled overtraining" and "structural training", to optimize your physiology and prepare your body for muscle growth. This book is for serious weight trainers who are ready to DEMOLISH plateaus and achieve growth and strength increases previously thought unattainable. Best of all, every training session is designed to be completed in less than an hour!

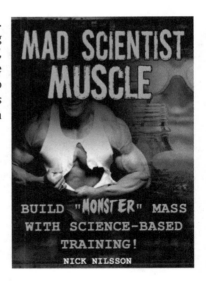

Also included:

- Detailed nutrition section
- Supplement guide
- Low-carb dieting option
- "Lazy Cook" muscle-building recipes

This book includes the most INSANELY effective training techniques you'll ever experience. It is packed with powerful training methods designed to build MASSIVE muscle by using a volume/intensity-driven format.